The Best-Kept Secret
to Raising a Healthy Child

CRAIG WEHRENBERG, D.C.
TRACEY MULHALL-WEHRENBERG, D.C.

Published by Specific Chiropractic
1673 Route 9, Clifton Park, New York 12065

Cover design by Kariann Wolf, Virtual Flow
Photography by Tom Stock, Stock Studios Photography
StopSIDS.org logo design and artwork on p. 12, 13 by Shawn Banner.
Cartoon on p. 18 used with permission by Peter Cranton, D.C.

Printed in the United States of America

ISBN 0-615-11485-7

Dedication

This book is dedicated to my brother Jeffrey Paul Wehrenberg and the precious infants who never had the opportunity to experience life to its fullest. Our thoughts and prayers are with all the families whose lives have been touched by the unfortunate and senseless passing of an infant.

CRAIG WEHRENBERG, D.C.

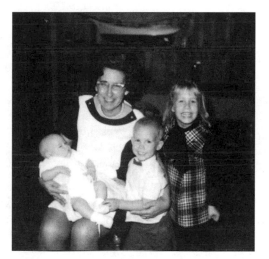

This is the last picture that I have of my brother, Jeffrey. On the back of the picture it reads,

Nov 27, 1969
Thanksgiving:
Grammy and her 3 Grandchildren

Little did anyone know that one month later, there would only be two grandchildren. Jeffrey died December 26, 1969.

Acknowledgments

We want to acknowledge several people who have influenced our lives and without whom the publishing of this book would not have been possible. First, we salute the many pioneers that laid the groundwork in chiropractic and gave us the profession we have today. These people endured suffering and persecution as they held true to their beliefs to help sick people get well. Without these visionaries, chiropractic would not have advanced to where it is today. Included in this list is, of course, Dr. B.J. Palmer, the developer of chiropractic who performed years of research on the spine.

Next, we thank the people who have influenced our lives both personally and professionally, especially Dr. Roy Sweat, whose dedication to our profession and to the Atlas Orthogonal organization is endless. We are not alone in saying, "This man has been like a father to us." We greatly appreciate his tireless efforts to improve our efficiency in correcting atlas vertebra subluxations. The late Dr. John D. Grostic was instrumental in the direction we have taken regarding research as he encouraged us in the Research Department at Life Chiropractic College. Dr. Lasca Hospers, our Research Advisor, led us to practice the Atlas Orthogonal procedure. Without these three key people, our lives would be on an entirely different path.

We would also like to thank our parents Ray and Margaret Wehrenberg and Harry and Lillian Mulhall whose endless support and encouragement have allowed us to follow our dreams, even when we were not understood by others. Other family members, friends and patients cannot be forgotten, as well, for their constant support of chiropractic and our beliefs.

We also wish to thank the National Sudden Infant Death Syndrome Resource Center for providing us with the many research abstracts used in this book.

Above all, we wish to thank and honor God, our creator and source of all life, who has given us this vision and the gift of healing as chiropractors so that we may touch, and change the lives of others to truly make a difference in this world.

Contents

Preface

This book was inspired by many years of research on Sudden Infant Death Syndrome (SIDS). Based on our research, we are convinced that the incidence of SIDS can be greatly reduced by taking a few simple, yet important steps in infant health that are currently overlooked. Although the ideas and concepts presented in this book may contradict traditional medical theories, which sometimes are referred to as "conventional wisdom," we believe they are ideas whose time has come. Conventional wisdom and accepted practices will not always give us the answers necessary to live life to its fullest. Once the ideas and theories that we will present are understood and stand up to the test of time and research, the current ideas of accepted and normal practices will change and many paradigms will shift regarding infant health.

We hope that the reader will come to understand the need for proper spinal maintenance for children. Once one truly understands the inherent, recuperative abilities of the body, what chiropractors refer to as "Innate Intelligence", then it will be easier to accept these beliefs. Just as good dental hygiene has become a common, every day practice, so should maintaining and properly caring for our spines. We believe until more natural, preventative health measures are practiced our nation's health will be plagued with serious, chronic illness. We envision a society free of dis-ease, where children and adults are well and fully in tune with the world around them. We have been encouraged by the words of our chiropractic forefather, Dr. B.J. Palmer who said,

> *We never know how far reaching something we may think, say or do today will affect the lives of millions tomorrow.*

What better time than now to tell the world, who desperately needs improved health, that chiropractic is a safe, effective method to unleash the powerful, innate healing capabilities of the human body?

We will donate a portion of the proceeds from the sale of this book to the non-profit foundation *StopSIDS.org*. This organization was created with the purpose of researching the impact of correcting spinal malfunction on infant health and SIDS. You can support the research efforts of *StopSIDS.org* by encouraging others to purchase this book, by visiting the Web site and sending a tax-deductible donation to: *StopSIDS.org*, 1673 Route 9, Suite 2, Clifton Park, NY, 12065.

As we were preparing to launch research projects through *StopSIDS.org* and write this book, we came across some people that discouraged us from doing this work. They told us that because SIDS *only* claims about 3,000 infant lives per year, not enough people would be interested in this project. Our reply was, "Well, it makes all the difference in the world to those 3,000 families that lose a child every year!"

We are reminded of the story where a little boy was running around the beach, throwing starfish that had washed up on the shore back into the ocean so that they would not dry out and die. As a passerby approached, he asked the little boy, "What are you doing?" The little boy picked up a starfish and threw it back into the ocean, saying, "I'm saving the lives of these starfish. Won't you help me?" The passerby said, "Don't be silly, the beach is covered with starfish. You can't possibly make a difference." The little boy picked up another and threw it back into the ocean as he said, "Well, I just made a difference to *that* one!" Having three children of our own, we know how special each individual baby is, and we believe we *can* make a difference in many infants' lives.

We are also reminded of the inspiring movie *Dead Poet's Society,* when Mr. Keating (Robin Williams) explained to the boys of his class,

> *The powerful play [of life] goes on and we all get to contribute a verse. What will your verse be? . . . Make your life extraordinary!*

Later in the movie, while standing on his desk, he asked his students, "Why do I stand on this desk?" The answer was, "Because we all need to see things differently once in a while." We believe this book and the *StopSIDS.org* research projects will be our *verse.* We hope that millions of people, as a result of this book, will begin to see things a little differently, and the health of many infants and children will be improved because of the work accomplished through the *StopSIDS.org Foundation.*

We understand that areas of this book will be difficult to read due to the tragic nature of SIDS as well as the details some of the research reports present. For this reason we apologize, especially to the families that have lost a child to SIDS. In no way do we wish to trivialize or re-open the pain that you have experienced. It is our hope, however, that by revealing the research information that we have assembled, family tragedies similar to yours might be avoided in the future and the health of many infants will be improved.

The theories, thoughts, ideas and beliefs in this book are ours alone and do not represent any particular chiropractic college, university, association, organization or foundation. Footnotes are used throughout the book, and the references can be found at the end of the book, to make reference and give credit to the source of research and theories of others where due.

CRAIG WEHRENBERG, D.C.
TRACEY MULHALL-WEHRENBERG, D.C.

Introduction

For over one hundred years, doctors of chiropractic have helped sick people become well. Yet, to most people this natural healing art is still a mystery, a secret. We are about to share with you the truth about the many benefits that chiropractic has to offer sick people. The beautiful expression of life, and the untapped potential in millions of human beings can be brought out with chiropractic. We hope you will come to understand this wonderful secret and the gift of health it holds.

The main goal of this book is to demonstrate how a misalignment of the atlas (the top vertebra in the spine) can cause infants' and children's health to suffer, and even cause death in some infants. We also want to increase the general public's understanding of how chiropractic, as it corrects these misalignments, can have a positive impact on children's health. Although we will make reference to SIDS and hope that we can reduce the incidence of this tragic syndrome, we intend to broaden our scope and look at all infant deaths, since many infant deaths do not fit into the SIDS definition.

Today in the United States there are approximately 3,000 deaths each year attributed to SIDS. According to the National SIDS Alliance more children die of SIDS in one year than all children (up to age fourteen) who die of cancer, heart disease, pneumonia, child abuse, AIDS, cystic fibrosis, and muscular dystrophy combined. During the past twenty-five years, over 100,000 families in the United States have had an infant die suddenly and unexpectedly of Sudden Infant Death Syndrome.

We would like to reduce the incidence of **all** infant deaths, which there are approximately 30,000 each year. Of course, we do not want to imply that we can save the life of every infant by adjusting the atlas, for there are many congenital diseases, deformities, birth traumas and other disorders that we obviously cannot help. It is our goal, however, to find a few pieces of the puzzle to SIDS and all infant deaths, and to help more babies experience optimum health and lead full, healthy lives.

Sudden infant death syndrome is a recognized medical disorder, one that is only diagnosed after the baby's death. By definition, the diagnosis is only given after investigation into the death of an infant fails to give an explanation of the death. What we hope to accomplish with this book and our research through the *StopSIDS.org* Foundation, is to reveal previously overlooked issues in infant health, primarily, the relationship between the upper neck and the nerve system and the impact this relationship has on health.

Atlas Orthogonality (AO for short) is a specialized chiropractic procedure which utilizes no manipulation and focuses on making structural corrections in the spine. These corrections are achieved by correcting misalignments in the upper neck, primarily the first vertebra in the spine, the atlas. This gentle, precise procedure of removing nerve system interference helps many people achieve improved health and find relief from a variety of symptoms, including neck and back pain, headaches, asthma, allergies, and many other health problems.

We are going to explain here what we believe is a main cause of ill health and death in many infants. We believe it is common for an infant to experience spinal trauma and have misalignments in the upper neck (primarily the atlas) before, during, or shortly after the birth process. The chiropractic profession calls these misalignments "subluxations" (pronounced sub luk-sa' shuns), which produce nerve system irritation. These misalignments may prevent the critical structures of the brain stem (which control the respiratory and cardiac centers) from maturing properly and to malfunction. This malfunction may cause an infant to either stop breathing and/or experience abnormal heart function. These two factors, alone *or* together, can cause an infant's health to suffer and may even cause an infant to succumb to this tragic syndrome we call SIDS. These misalignments can also lower the body's immune function and an infant's resistance to illness and infection. This decreased functioning immune system can leave an infant susceptible to infections, which may also lead to a senseless death.

Researchers before us have suggested a connection between spinal subluxations and SIDS. For the purpose of this book and our research, we call this connection the Atlas VSC-SIDS Theory. VSC stands for Vertebral Subluxation Complex, which means one or more segments of the spine (including the joints at the base of the head) are not positioned correctly and cause the nerve system to malfunction. We will get into much greater detail in Chapter Four, but briefly, when the atlas vertebra (the top vertebra of the spine) is misaligned, *at least* three different complications can take place that may lead to decreased health and SIDS:

1) Spinal cord and brain stem distortion (minor stretching or compromise)

2) Electrical and chemical signals to and from the brain get "confused"

3) Blood supply to the brain stem and other critical areas of the brain may be decreased, resulting in hypoxia (lack of oxygen to this area) through:

   A. Vertebral artery ischemia (lack of blood flowing through the arteries that travel up through openings in the neck and supply the brain stem and other vital nerve centers)

   B. Venous blood pooling (blood in the veins in this area not draining properly)

There is a syndrome associated with the atlas vertebral subluxation complex, which is called the Atlas Neuro-Vascular Syndrome (ANVS), a term first coined by Dr. Jeffry Finnigan in his book *Life Beyond Headaches*. As the name implies, when an atlas subluxation is present, there are both nerve system and vascular disturbances which can lead to a decrease in one's overall health potential.

The rest of this book (primarily supported by scientific medical research) will explain why we feel so strongly about the Atlas VSC-SIDS Theory. As questions come up in your mind about the validity of this theory, please keep in mind some facts that are common medical knowledge:

1) The brain stem *is* the primary control center for breathing and heart functions.

2) The vagus nerve originates in the brain stem and affects many areas such as the heart, lungs, stomach, ears, pharynx, larynx, trachea, esophagus, and the majority of the autonomic (automatic) functions and internal organs.

3) These critical neurological structures (the brain stem and the vagus nerve) are closely connected to the atlas vertebra.

4) Many scientific research studies have shown a connection between the brain stem and SIDS.

One of our research goals is to investigate whether dysfunction at the brain stem can be improved through specific chiropractic adjustments of the atlas; and improve neurological function. The belief system that chiropractors have adhered to for over one hundred years is that when nerve interference is removed through spinal adjustments, the body is allowed to function at 100%, enabling the body to express its optimum level of health.

We have one request for you as you read this book: ***please*** keep an open mind. We have been very encouraged over the past few years with the trend in our nation towards the exploration of, and in some cases, the acceptance of so-called "alternative medicine," such as chiropractic. In the *Journal of the American Medical Association* it was reported that in 1997, Americans made more visits to alternative practitioners than to traditional medical doctors. We have many people to thank for this trend and we feel it is primarily due to the fact that we as a society are becoming more educated about how our bodies work and are taking more responsibility in the care of them. People are beginning to realize that it makes more sense to help keep the body healthy, instead of just treating symptoms. For over one hundred years, chiropractors have been saying, "Health comes from within: from Above-Down, Inside-Out" (from the brain, through the spinal cord and nerves, to cells and tissues), and it is apparent that this philosophy is proving to be the case.

1

Spinal Compromise Before and During Birth as a Cause of Atlas misalignment (Atlas VSC)

While the birth process is a wondrous time, and many babies appear to be delivered in good health, the final stages of development in the womb, and the subsequent journey into the world, can have damaging effects on a newborn's spine. Whether cramped by uterine or abdominal constraints before the birth process begins, or by being twisted or stretched in the trip down and out of the birth canal, many newborns have misalignments in their spines, which cause nerve interference (VSC). Our research suggests that this interference can lead to SIDS, and at the very least, abnormal growth and development producing sub-optimum health conditions through childhood and beyond.

Pre-Birth Spinal Compromise

As the fetus fills out the uterus in the last ten weeks of pregnancy, the volume ratio of the fetus to amniotic fluid becomes progressively increased. If the fetus is mal-positioned as the cushion of fluid decreases, this puts the fetus at risk for bone and soft tissue malformation and can produce a VSC before birth.

Doctors Dunne and Clarren in their paper, "The Origin of Prenatal and Postnatal Deformities," stated:

> *'Deformations' or 'deformities' are anomalies that ensue when tissues are dis-*

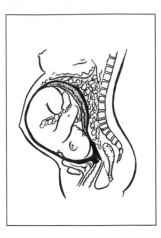

Uterine constraint can take place during the last few months while the fetus is developing in the womb. If a fetus is mal-positioned in the womb, he or she can be susceptible to spinal compromise (VSC) and malformations.

torted through abnormal mechanical forces. The musculoskeletal system is especially susceptible to deformity. Unlike other types of dysmorphogenesis [congenital malformations], all of which originate prenatally, deformations may occur before or after birth .[1]

In layman's terms, certain congenital or inherited defects occur before birth, but deformations of the spine and other muscles and bones can occur in utero or after the birth process.

The authors went on to explain how biomechanical forces are important to the proper development of muscles, ligaments, cartilage, and bone. They agreed with many other authors who believed that constraint in the uterus can cause deformities seen at birth. We believe these deformities or malformations in the spine causing VSC, can lead to damaging nerve interference.

Uterine constraint is more likely in first-born infants when the uterine muscle tone is at its greatest, in the unusually large fetus or if there is a decreased amount of amniotic fluid. Additional constraint may be generated within the uterus or in the abdominal or pelvic cavities. Intrauterine space-occupying bodies such as additional fetuses, a bicornuate uterus [a uterus that is a variation from normal, that has two horns, or cornua], or uterine fibroids may restrict fetal movement. Extrauterine compression may originate from tight abdominal musculature, especially in first pregnancies, or from bony maternal structures such as a prominent lumbar spine or a small pelvis and small stature. Maternal hypertension has also been significantly associated with fetal deformation, but the mechanism is unknown.

Basically what Dunne and Clarren were saying was that abnormal uterine constraint and other factors can produce abnormal stress on the infant's spine even before delivery. This means an infant can have spinal compromise (a vertebral subluxation complex) before the birth process even begins.

They also stated:

While many postnatal deformities can be contained or corrected by the application of counteracting forces, aggressive physical therapy, casting, or surgery is often required for correction.

We suggest that conservative chiropractic, focusing on atlas adjusting (correction) should be the first method of correction employed in these infants with postnatal deformities. In our opinion many deformities are mislabeled as "congenital" but were actually caused by uterine constraint or birth trauma. If corrected early, before the bones and soft tissue become molded, they can be prevented. We have seen several cases of infant torticollis, where the infant could not straighten his or her head due to neck muscle spasms, respond well to atlas correction.

Spinal Subluxation During Labor & Delivery

If the infant gets through the pregnancy without compromise to the spine, it is not uncommon that labor and delivery will cause a subluxation. Dr. Joseph Flesia stated, "We now have over 100 references indicating that the Vertebral Subluxation Complex can happen at the birth process or early in life." [2] Dr. Larry Webster stated, "New studies are now indicating that the birth process may be one of the foremost causes of Vertebral Subluxation." [3]

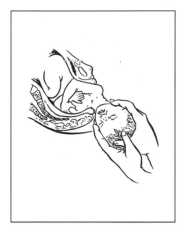

This is an illustration of a baby being delivered from the birth canal. Doctors are taught to traction the neck to assist the delivery of the first shoulder, and then pull the head the other way to get the second shoulder out. If the infant is having a difficult time coming out, it does not take a lot of force from the attendant (doctor or mid-wife) to cause an Atlas VSC.

Birth, even under optimum conditions, is a very traumatic process.[4] Post-natal investigations, especially computer-tomographic research, has shaken the view that normal birth is a problem-free event.[5] During active labor, the spine is particularly exposed to injury as it is forced through the birth canal; this is especially so if the birth is a rapid one. The spinal nerve roots at birth are prone to injury by the maneuver of bringing the shoulder down by lateral traction on the head. This puts great stress on the brachial plexus (a complex system of nerves coming from the middle and lower neck) and spinal nerve roots, and is a common cause of Erb's palsy and Klumpke's paralysis (two different paralyses involving the arms).[4]

Certain obstetrical situations tend to put the newborn at an increased risk of a traumatic birth. These situations include, but are not limited to, a very fast delivery, premature delivery, breech delivery, and cesarean delivery. Even the skilled hand of the obstetrician or midwife may apply extreme force, traction, and torsion to the cervical spine of the newborn resulting in an Atlas Vertebral Subluxation Complex (VSC) and causing Atlas Neuro-Vascular Syndrome.

The use of vacuum extractors and forceps to remove the infant from the birth canal have been known to apply extreme forces and place a new born at risk of injury.[6-26] Dr. Towner, in a paper that he wrote with three other researchers, stated:

> *Infants delivered by vacuum extraction or other operative techniques may be more likely to sustain major injuries than those delivered spontaneously, but the extent of the risk is unknown.*[27]

The researchers reported that the incidence of death associated with spontaneous vaginal delivery was 1 per 5000. However, when the vacuum extractor was used, the death rate jumped to 1 per 3333 and with forceps delivery it was even worse, at 1 per 2000 births. They also reported that the incidence of intracranial hemorrhage (bleeding in the brain) associated with spontaneous delivery was 1 per 1900, with vacuum extraction delivery it was 1 per 860, and with forceps delivery it was a staggering 1 per 664 births. Towner and others found the combination of vacuum extraction and forceps delivery significantly increased the risks of brain and connective tissue hemorrhage to 1 per 277 births. Facial-nerve injury, and brachial plexus (nerves coming from the neck) injury were also increased. This combination also increased the risk of convulsions to 1 per 400 births. They also pointed out that a cesarean section performed after a failed attempt at vaginal delivery with the use of one of these devices is also associated with a significant increased risk of injury. Specifically, when the head has been pulled by forceps or vacuum extractor, but failed to deliver the baby, then c-section was performed, the risk of intracranial hemorrhage was 1 per 333 births and the risk of convulsions was increased to 1 per 142 births.

The article was published in the December 1999 issue of the *New England Journal of Medicine* and provoked several letters to the editor in reply. One such letter was written by Aldo Vacca, M.B., B.S., who stated:

> *The report by Towner et al. should be read by all obstetricians who use vacuum extraction. If they are not persuaded to review the practice of vacuum extraction in the face of the evidence of harm to the infants, as presented by Towner et al., I doubt that any form of persuasion will ever be effective.*[28]

The vacuum extractor looks like a suction cup that fits on the infant's skull, then is pressurized and used to pull the baby out. Forceps look like salad tongs and are used to grip the baby's head, then twist and pull it out of the birth canal. An article in the April 2000 *Obstetrics and Gynecology Journal* reported an overall incidence in the use of forceps and vacuum extraction to be 9.2%, and that the rate decreased from 12.6% in 1992 to 6.9% in 1999.[29] It may just be a coincidence, but it is interesting to note the rate of SIDS also decreased by similar percentages over the course of those years.

A word of advice for parents that have infants that were delivered with either the vacuum extractor or forceps: please take your baby to a doctor of chiropractic and ask them to examine your baby's spine, particularly the upper cervical spine. Studies have shown that infants that appear healthy may have suffered birth trauma that has gone undiagnosed.[30] We believe this undiagnosed birth trauma can have life changing effects on children and spinal misalignments need to be corrected early in infants to achieve optimum health.

Another factor that warrants close examination is whether the labor and delivery was an extended one, exposing the infant's spine to increased stress due to prolonged uterine contractions. Try to visualize what takes place as the mother's uterus contracts, it squeezes the infant downward, compressing its head, neck and spine as it approaches and finally passes through the birth canal. In particularly long labors, this can put a tremendous amount of compressional force on the cervical spine, causing it to become subluxated.

An infant delivered in the breech position is at an increased risk of spinal trauma and subluxations due to the variation in positioning. Dr. Abroms reported that **seventy-five percent of infants born in the breech position with hyperextension of the head exhibit spinal cord injury**. [31] Dr. Painter also reported a significant amount of spinal cord injury associated with breech deliveries. [32]

Stretching Forces

Injuries to the spinal cord generally occur as a result of torsional (twisting) and longitudinal (lengthening) stretching forces.[4] It must be noted that the vertebral arteries travel through the foramina transversarii (outlets) of the upper six cervical vertebrae, and hence spinal distortion with injury to these vessels may result in ischemia (deficiency of blood due to interruption of blood supply) of the cervical cord and brain stem.

Drs. Anrig and Forrester in their book, *The Peter Pan Potential* refer to the research paper "Latent Spinal Cord and Brainstem Injury in Newborn Infants" by Abraham Towbin, as follows:

> *Perhaps the most important paper in contemporary literature substantiating the absolute necessity for all children to receive chiropractic care immediately following the birth process.* [33]

In his paper, Dr. Towbin reviewed the significance of brain stem and upper spinal cord injury at birth and their manifestations of symptoms, from mild inflammatory responses to shock, with disturbance of respiratory and other vital functions leading to death. Towbin emphasized that the primary cause of neonatal spinal injury is forceful, excessive longitudinal traction, particularly when combined with flexion of the spinal axis during delivery. Two mechanisms of brain stem damage are stretch-injury and compression-injury. He stated:

> *The force of traction applied during delivery may be transmitted upward, affecting the brainstem. Deep stretch-injury may occur, resulting in major tears and hemorrhage. Forceful traction tends to produce compression injury to the brain stem by the medulla [the lowest section of the brain stem] being drawn into the foramen magnum [the opening at the base of the skull that the spinal cord travels through]. This mechanism can be demonstrated in the infant at autopsy. The lower brainstem throttled in the foramen magnum, is subject to surface injury as well as compression.*[34]

In the case of cephalic (head first) presentation where spinal cord injury is present, the damage is usually sustained from torsional forces. In these cases the injury is usually above the brachial connection of the spinal cord (above the middle of the neck).

Dr. Towbin described six cases that had a difficult birth and sustained birth trauma. All cases died anywhere from two to seventeen hours after birth.[35]

Please don't think the answer to birth trauma is in cesarean-section deliveries. It has been shown that infants born via c-section have abnormally lower blood pressure measurements than babies born vaginally.[36] Studies have also found that infants delivered by c-section have a lower metabolic activity of certain immune factors, which may leave this child more susceptible to infections.[37] Another study found that elective, repeat cesarean section often leads to respiratory distress syndrome (RDS) in infants.[38]

Atlas Instability (a feature of the VSC) Implicated in SIDS

In 1979 a landmark, painstaking study that supports the Atlas VSC-SIDS Theory was conducted by Dr. Floyd Gilles and others at the Children's Hospital Medical Center in Boston.[39] The researchers examined twenty-two infants, ranging in age from 0 to 26 months, that had recently died. Five of the infant cadavers were not dissected. The other seventeen (eleven SIDS and six non-SIDS) underwent x-ray and dissection studies of the upper cervical spine. The results of this study were dramatic! The researchers found that atlas instability (a feature of VSC) was implicated in SIDS.

To summarize three of the most important findings:

- All of the seventeen infants that were autopsied had spinal malformations, whether their death was diagnosed as SIDS or not.

- In ten of the infants, extension of the head created an indentation on the brain stem, which was caused by the atlas (C-1). We believe this instability of the atlas that caused the brain stem insult is the result of a mal-positioned atlas (VSC).

- In five infants, vertebral artery angiograms were successfully performed. Three out of the five demonstrated vertebral artery compression during extension of the head. It was later discovered that these three also had atlas instability (a feature of atlas VSC). The two that did not have vertebral artery compression did not have atlas instability. The vertebral arteries run through the atlas vertebra on both sides and supply the blood to the brain stem. It stands to reason that a subluxation or misalignment of the atlas can cause these critical arteries to malfunction. This is one reason why Atlas VSC incorporates Atlas Neuro-Vascular Syndrome, since the misalignment not only causes neurological compromise, but also vascular (blood flow) compromise.

The findings in Gilles' study are too significant to blame strictly on coincidence and present strong support that the Atlas VSC-SIDS Theory should be closely examined, and intensely researched. Methods must be tested to determine what can be done to correct atlas instability in infants. We believe the Atlas Orthogonal Procedure is one of the safest, most effective methods of removing damaging misalignments that can cause atlas instability and nerve system interference.

Two of our mentors, Dr. Roy Sweat and Dr. Lasca Hospers were involved in a study by the Association for Research in Chiropractic Sciences (ARCS) that was designed to test Gilles' findings. The ARCS study agreed with the findings of Gilles. This study was a triple blind research project that involved x-ray analysis of fifty deceased infants. The researchers found that **all cases of atlas inversion were SIDS cases**, but not all SIDS cases exhibited atlas inversion. This finding supports what the Atlas VSC-SIDS Theory suggests: the Atlas VSC can cause SIDS, but there are other causes as well. This important study emphasizes the need for infants to be examined by a chiropractor, specifically in the atlas area, shortly after their birth. The authors stated,

> . . . *relative measurements suggested that a correlation existed between instability in the atlanto-occipital articulation and Sudden Infant Death Syndrome.*[40]

Upper cervical instability along with atlas inversion into the foramen magnum can cause incomplete or temporary compromise to the blood supply of the upper spinal cord and brain stem. This can cause impairment of the respiratory centers in the medulla (brain stem) as seen in "chronic intermittent hypoxia" (long-term decrease in oxygen) present at autopsies of SIDS cases.[40] Dr. Hospers and others stated:

> *This mechanism may also be the causal agent with infants that have other conventional diseases.*

They went on to quote Gilles:

> *At this early stage in the development of our notions about the potential contribution of atlanto-occipital instability to deaths in infants, it is very difficult to assess the role of this proposed mechanism in the death of an infant with a conventional disease. Thus, one might anticipate that the 'controls' will be contaminated by children who had a conventional disease, but whose death was in fact, caused by this mechanism."*

They stated *"In other words, an infant who died of a 'conventional disease' may have actually died from the effects of atlas inversion.*

We hypothesize that due to abnormal positioning in the womb, an infant's upper neck can become deformed and render him or her susceptible to compromise of the brain stem and other critical neuroanatomy in this area. Since the infant's spine is not totally molded at the time of birth, birth trauma or abnormal stress and tension on the neck during the birth process can also lead to the deformities seen in the two previously mentioned studies. It is our hope that through early examination, detection and proper treatment of the upper neck, these children will be able to live healthy lives.

With the help of Drs. Sweat and Hospers, we have plans for research projects that will study Atlas VSC and its correction in infants. We believe that if the atlas subluxations in infants are identified and corrected, these infants will have a much better chance for a healthy life.

The Difficulty of Recognizing Post-Delivery Spinal Cord & Brain Stem Injury

We have one major concern as more infants are brought to doctors of chiropractic for examination and care. This concern is that there may be spinal cord and brain stem injuries present in the infant that took place in the birth process that may be so severe that correction of the atlas subluxation may not be enough to allow the infant to live a normal healthy life. Often, this injury is misdiagnosed, as a paper from the division of Neurosurgery at Duke University Medical Center in 1992 pointed out. In four out of the five cases the researchers presented, spinal cord trauma was misdiagnosed by the referring physicians, including pediatric neurologists.[41]

Since the spinal cord is relatively inelastic when compared with the surrounding vertebral canal, vertebral fracture or subluxation may not necessarily be visible with spinal cord and brain stem trauma.[4] In other words, injury to the soft tissue nerve structures may be present without visible damage to the spine.

We believe it is in the best interest of the infant to have a spinal examination for VSC even if there is serious neurological damage. Again, when there are no subluxations present, an individual has a greater chance of experiencing optimum health, regardless of the condition they present with. This may place the chiropractor in a more precarious position, as infants may be presented to a doctor of chiropractic in a vulnerable (damaged) state. However, if safe, noninvasive adjusting procedures are used, such as the Atlas Orthogonal Procedure, there is very little chance of causing any harm to an infant's spine or nerve system.

Healthy Infants—Why They Need an Atlas Examination

We would like to emphasize the point that many seemingly healthy infants have vertebral subluxations that occurred before, during, or shortly after the birth process that go undetected. In 1992, Dr. H. Biedermann wrote an article that was published in the German Medical Journal, *Medicine,* in which he quoted a research study of one thousand seemingly health infants. It was discovered that eleven percent of these infants had "atlas blockages," what we would call an atlas VSC. Upon further investigation, seventy-eight percent of those babies had asymmetries of the spine, such as scoliotic curvature. He stated,

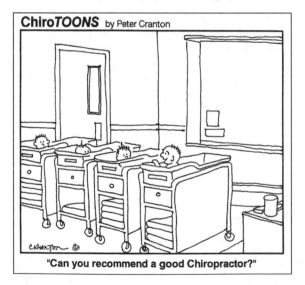

ChiroTOONS by Peter Cranton

"Can you recommend a good Chiropractor?"

We can safely assume that most of these children would not have been considered in need of a treatment had they not been included in this study. Six percent of British primary school children have significant disorders of their visuomotor system. How many of these could profit from manual therapy of the suboccipital joints [an atlas adjustment]?[42]

As we mentioned earlier, studies have shown that infants that appear healthy may have suffered birth trauma that has gone undiagnosed. Researchers from the Department of Neurology, at the Medical University of South Carolina, found that **half** of the infants they studied that were delivered without complication had small masses of blood accumulation in different areas of the brain. On follow-up examination, all children appeared to show "normal" growth and development.[30] A chiropractic examination may have shown otherwise, since a medical examination does not identify the vertebral subluxation complex. In other words, although these children appeared to have "normal" growth and development according to the traditional medical model, from a chiropractic perspective, they most likely would have been diagnosed with a misalignment in their spine which is undetectable by the human eye and which can subtly alter their health potential.

The previous research reports should help the general public understand why we recommend that **all infants should have their atlas examined shortly after birth,** since half of the infants studied that appeared to be born without complication demonstrated nerve system compromise.

The German medical doctor, Gottfried Gutmann in his paper "Blocked Atlantal Nerve Syndrome in Infants and Small Children" stressed the importance of having an infant's neck examined as well. He believes that the majority of newborns are born with micro trauma in the area of the brain stem, which we believe is a result of Atlas VSC and Atlas Neuro-Vascular Syndrome. He stated:

> *In the majority of newborn children, microparenchymic injuries [micro-trauma] of the brain-segments near the ventricle have been found. Other investigators more often confirmed a distortion of the head-neck connection.*[43]

The board of directors of *StopSIDS.org* and the doctors that have agreed to participate in the important research studies are excited about what the next few years will reveal about atlas adjusting and its impact on infant health. We believe it will show that by correcting atlas subluxations, a profound positive impact on health and vitality will result.

Chiropractic Care and Its Impact on Childhood Health

In order to understand the ramifications of chiropractic treatment on infants we must first review relevant anatomy and chiropractic tenets. The Glossary includes important definitions for relevant parts of the anatomy. A quick review of it is recommended before reading further.

What is Chiropractic?

Chiropractic was founded on the hypothesis that a spinal misalignment, or Vertebral Subluxation Complex (VSC) interferes with normal nerve transmission to tissue cells and alters normal function. Dr. Palmer proved this hypothesis in the 1930's with the use of the electroencephaloneuromentimpograph (timpograph).[1] Basically, the timpograph measured nerve impulses at different spinal levels. Dr. Palmer found that when a decrease in normal nerve transmission was detected and a subluxation present, it could be improved by giving a specific spinal adjustment. Presently these findings are being repeated with more sophisticated equipment such as somatosensory evoked potentials[2-4] and surface electrode electromyography.[5] These are specialized tests that measure the electrical signals as they travel from nerves and muscles to the brain.

In the simplest of terms, for over 100 years chiropractors have been saying the nerve system is *the* controlling factor in our bodies and greatly affects our health. Since the spine houses the nerve system, when a vertebra is out of alignment (subluxated), this causes interference to the proper function of the nerve system, thus disrupting the communication between the brain and the body. This miscommunication, or short-circuiting can cause some part of one's health to suffer. When a misaligned vertebra is restored to its proper position through a chiropractic adjustment, the nerve system interference is removed and proper function is restored.

The vertebral subluxation complex has been written about and researched by many doctors. The vertebral subluxation complex has five components: abnormal spinal motion, abnormal nerve function, abnormal muscle function, abnormal cellular changes, and spinal and systemic degeneration and disorders. Therefore it is easy to understand how a VSC can have negative effects on one's overall health because a VSC can affect spinal motion, nerve and muscle function and integrity and has an effect on the cells of the body. We believe the atlas vertebral subluxation complex is the most important entity that robs people of their health. The removal of the Atlas VSC is the **best-kept secret** and the key to optimum health.

What is Health?

How would you answer the question, "What is Health?"

Dorland's Medical Dictionary says health is,

> *The optimal state of physical, mental and social well-being and not merely the absence of disease and infirmity.*

So, health is not how we feel. For instance, if a man feels great and goes into his doctor's office for a check-up and the doctor tells him he has six months to live due to inoperable, terminal cancer, was that man sick or well the day before? Obviously, he was sick. Now let's say another man eats some food that has spoiled, and gets violently ill with vomiting and diarrhea. Is that man sick or well? (Trick question, isn't it?) He is having a healthy response. The body recognized the toxins in the food and wanted to get them out of his system through all possible means. Therefore, he should thank his body for responding in such a manner. Similarly, a fever is the body's way of burning unwanted pathogens in our body and is a healthy response.

Chiropractic and Health

Do you think chiropractors primarily treat for back pain, headaches, and neck pain? Today many people do. Since 1895 chiropractors have been getting excellent results with these types of symptoms and *many* more. Because we work on the spine, and get excellent results with spine and other musculoskeletal symptoms, many people have associated chiropractic with pain relief. We have advertised that we can help with these symptoms, primarily because *we do*. Numerous research studies have been performed that show the effectiveness of chiropractic care in relieving pain and dis-comfort as well as being cost-effective.

There is however, so much more to chiropractic than just the treatment of pain. Chiropractors work on the spine. The spine houses the nerve system, which controls *everything* in the body. There is not a system, organ, tissue or cell in the body that can operate without proper nerve supply. The body has an amazing innate intelligence that functions through the nerve system to maintain health and homeostasis in the body. If you were to spend some time in our office, you would think chiropractors treat just about everything. There are people that have come in that had horrible asthma and now do not need their inhalers anymore. There are children that used to have ear infections whose medical doctor wanted to put tubes in their ears; we adjusted them and now they don't suffer from the ear infections. Other children had bed-wetting problems and now they wake up with dry sheets. Other people had migraines and now they are headache free. Have we lost you yet? Here is the point that we need you to understand: Chiropractors don't "treat" or "cure" anything . . . the body heals itself, as long as there is no nerve interference! All we do as chiropractors is remove the nerve interference and allow the body to function more efficiently. Chiropractic is the original mind (brain)—body connection profession.

It is our belief that newborns' health can be improved by ensuring their spines are properly aligned. We understand that many people will not immediately accept our theories and suggestions that all infants should have an atlas examination by a doctor of chiropractic as soon as possible after birth. We understand that the present paradigm held by many people is that chiropractors are primarily for neck, back and other musculoskeletal pain syndromes. However, just as many great thinkers and visionaries in history were ahead of their time, we believe it is just a matter of time before chiropractors are invited into hospitals to examine newborns shortly after delivery. We may not see this in our generation, but we believe it will take place someday.

Imagine if Christopher Columbus listened to his critics when they told him he was crazy because they (the "experts") *knew* the earth was flat and he was going to fall off in his pursuit for the New World. These members of the "Flat Earth Society" were the educated individuals in society, not just commoners. Similarly, some people may choose to believe the stereotypical thinking that chiropractors are effective only for back problems and that these thoughts regarding infant health that we are presenting are crazy. But remember—**history repeats itself! We are setting sail for a New World of infant health, despite any skeptics.**

Spinal Hygiene vs. Dental Hygiene: Which is more important?

The dental profession has done a wonderful job in raising awareness of the importance of dental hygiene. For decades, dentists have visited our children in the schools and taught them (as they chewed on those little red pills) to brush their teeth at least twice each day. Dental hygiene habits in America have forever been altered. We now know that we should floss daily and see our dentist regularly for cleanings starting at an early age. Our improved dental health can be traced back to the vigilant educational efforts of thousands of dentists.

Chiropractors have a similar responsibility when it comes to educating the public on proper spinal care. In fact, chiropractors have *more* of a responsibility due to the critical role the spine plays in relation to the nerve system and health. We have not found a class on spinal hygiene in any school health books to date. Think of the injustice being done to the public due to the lack of awareness. Ignorance is *not* bliss, and what you don't know *can* hurt you. Just think how little our children are taught about the nerve system and how it regulates our health. A decaying tooth can be replaced, but your spine is irreplaceable and your health depends on it. Children *and* parents need to be educated on the important role the spine plays regarding health.

In her paper "Physical Stresses of Childhood that could Lead to the Need for Chiropractic Care," presented at the first National Conference on Chiropractic and Pediatrics, in San Diego, California in 1991, Dr. Maxine McMullen stated:

> *Any condition that arises to change the normal birth process . . . frequently results in subluxation at the level of greatest stress. Severe subluxation resulting in nerve damage may be clinically obvious at birth (e.g. Bell's, Erb's, and Klumpke's palsies), however more frequently the trauma remains subclinical with symptoms arising at a later time. These symptoms include, but are not limited to irritability, colic, failure-to-thrive syndromes, and those syndromes associated with lowered immune responses. These subluxations should be analyzed and corrected as soon as possible after birth to prevent these associated conditions.*[7]

If every infant had the opportunity to be examined for Atlas VSC and ANVS, we believe that many tragic deaths would be avoided and many children would grow up healthier without unnecessary drugs and surgery. It is disturbing to look at the statistics of how many children are on prescription medications today. Many of the symptoms that are being treated, such as hyperactivity have been shown to improve under chiropractic care.[8, 9]

More research needs to be done along the lines of the study we were involved with as Research Assistants at Life Chiropractic College in 1989. The research was presented at the International Chiropractors Association Annual Conference in Tampa, Florida in 1990 by our research advisor, Dr. Lasca Hospers. The paper was titled, "Electroencephalographic observations of Children with Petit Mal and Petit Mal/Grand Mal Variant Epilepsies Before and After Life Upper Cervical Adjustment." The paper discussed three case studies of children with petit mal epilepsy (absent seizures) with and without grand mal combinations. The children ranged from five to twelve years of age. All three children were examined using electroencephalographic (EEG) recordings before and after atlas adjustment. By using specialized adjustment procedures in the upper neck, a positive effect on the brain stem was achieved; we were able to see a positive change through EEG recordings.

The details in the study were as follows. All three cases responded favorably to the atlas adjustments, although a chemical or post-traumatic lesion remained in two of the cases and moved in one of the cases. In the paper Dr. Hospers said,

> *Regardless of whether the lesion was permanent or changing, it appears that relieving pressure on the caudal brainstem ascending facilatory and inhibitory pathways and perhaps reducing interference with vertebral circulation by adjusting these critical segments, protected "normal" tissue.*

She concluded that,

> *Within the scope of visual EEG analysis, the Life Upper Cervical type of instrument adjusting appears to reduce invasiveness from regions of abnormal cortical activity and normalize and restore bilateral symmetry to normal tissue between seizure activity.*[10]

This limited paper of three cases showed that chiropractic adjustments could do the same thing that some of the anti-seizure drugs do, which is to reduce the spike component and protect surrounding tissue from invasion of it. Isn't it much better to have children under safe, effective chiropractic care than to have them on drugs with major side effects? We understand that drugs may be necessary at times, but should be a last resort, after all conservative approaches have been used.

Many Conditions Benefit from Chiropractic

Since the idea we present of **examining infants for atlas vertebral subluxations shortly after birth** is going to take many people by surprise, we want to supply you with some additional research that helps support our theories. There are many studies that show chiropractic treatment has helped to improve a variety of symptoms and diseases. Even *Dear Abby* published a column on the effectiveness of chiropractic treatment on bedwetting. As one of her readers wrote after the successful chiropractic treatment of her 15-year-old bed-wetting twin sons,

> . . . *there is a certain part of the spinal column that regulates the bladder— I can't explain it very well—but all I can say is it worked, which meant every- thing in the world to me and my boys.*

Many chiropractors who have treated children have successfully alleviated bed-wetting conditions. The explanation is a simple one: the nerve system controls every tissue, cell and organ in the body including the bladder. If the nerves that control the bladder are not functioning properly, then the bladder simply won't function properly either. When the misalignment in the spine is corrected and proper nerve flow is restored, the bladder is able to function as intended.

It is apparent through other published reports that chiropractic care can be helpful in such diverse disorders as cerebral palsy, seizure disorders, ear infections and others.[11-16] In fact a study published in 1996 demonstrated that ninety-three percent (93%) of the forty-six children studied with ear infections improved. Seventy-five percent (75%) of the children improved in ten days or less and forty-three percent (43%) improved with only one or two treatments.[17] Another study that was published in 1996 demonstrated a one hundred percent (100%) improvement in five cases with chronic ear infections.[18]

One study published in *The American Chiropractor*, titled "A Comparative Study of Health Status of Children Raised Under the Health Care Models of Chiropractic & Allopathic Medicine"[19] proved to be very interesting. This study showed that children raised under chiropractic care are less prone to infectious processes such as otitis media (middle ear infections) and tonsillitis, and that their immune systems are better able to cope with allergens such as pollen, weeds, grasses, etc. as compared to children raised under allopathic (traditional medical) care. The study also found that there was a significantly reduced use of antibiotic therapy among the chiropractic group; this indicated a lower susceptibility to bacterial infections as a result of greater immune system response. It was also noted that the children in the chiropractic group had a more rapid recovery period from injury or illness than other children their age.

The chiropractic community does not claim to treat or cure these or other symptoms. Rather, a doctor of chiropractic examines spines, to locate and remove vertebral subluxations to allow homeostasis in the body to prevail. We recognize that nerve interference can exist, and when it does, it disrupts normal health. As chiropractors, we simply remove the interference to normal health, by putting the spine back in place.

Can Chiropractic Adjustments Affect the Brain Stem?

For the purpose of this book and showing that chiropractic, through adjusting an infant's atlas, can help in the prevention of SIDS, we feel it is important to establish that chiropractic can help with abnormal brain and brain stem function.

The Brain Stem is *the* Control Center

The brain stem is the most critical area of the brain. Every message that is transmitted from the brain to the body and vice versa must go through this area. The brain stem greatly affects all the organs of the body, including those critical to life and health, such as the heart and lungs.

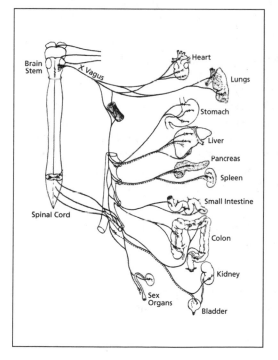

The illustration to the left demonstrates the importance of the brain stem and the nerves that come from this area, specifically the Vagus nerve. As you can see the brain stem has an effect on all the major organs of the body, including the heart and lungs."

In an article published in the *Journal of Behavioral Optometry*,[20] Doctors Gilman and Bergstrand describe the case of a 75-year-old male who had lost his vision following a traumatic injury to his neck. After being evaluated by an ophthalmologist, the clinical impression was that no treatment was indicated and the vision loss was permanent. The patient then sought treatment by Dr. Bergstrand, a chiropractor who diagnosed him with cervical subluxation and autonomic nervous system involvement. After the patient's third chiropractic adjustment his vision began returning, slowly at first and then to the point where he could read comfortably.

The patient, the chiropractor (Dr. Bergstrand) and the optometrist (Dr. Gilman) believed his vision returned due to the chiropractic treatments and not spontaneous remission. The authors give two suggestions for theories that could explain the return of vision; with the first being a connection between the spinal nerves of the upper cervical spine and the various visual fibers:

> *The connection is as follows: the first four cervical nerves communicate with the Rami communicants; the Rami communicants communicate with the superior cervical ganglion; the superior cervical ganglion communicates with the cavernous plexus (internal carotid nerve); the cavernous plexus communicates with the ciliary ganglion, the oculomotor nerve, the ophthalmic branch of the trigeminal nerve and the ophthalmic artery. Chiropractic theory indicates that physical interference with nerves can potentially cause dimunition of their function. In this case, chiropractic manipulation may have eliminated the interference with resulting return of visual function.*

> *A second theory to explain the return of vision would involve cervical soft tissue trauma (cervical subluxation complex) that affects the sympathetic innervation to the blood vessels of the optic nerve. By eliminating innervational interference, the optic nerve blood supply may have returned to normal after being constricted by the trauma.*

In simpler terms, a series of messages traveling through the nervous system control vision. When these messages are subjected to interference, vision may be impaired. Similarly, when nerve interference is eliminated, these nerves have a better chance of functioning normally. The blood supply may also return to normal and in the case of the optic nerve, vision can return to a more normal state. And so it is with many symptoms, syndromes and diseases. **The body can only function as well as the nervous system allows it to**. In chiropractic we do not treat these various symptoms, syndromes and diseases, but rather we remove the interference to the nervous system and allow the body to regain normal function. Chiropractic is as simple as that!

There have been several other studies published that reported improved vision following chiropractic treatment. One study from Australia described a 53-year-old woman who lost her vision three weeks after falling down a stairwell. She had two medical tests that showed she had optic nerve damage in both eyes, the right was worse than the left. After a course of chiropractic treatment (twenty visits) her vision had recovered. Another test was performed that demonstrated her optic nerve function had improved as well.[21]

Another paper that showed positive results from chiropractic treatment of seizures was published in 1990 in *The Journal of Chiropractic Research and Clinical Investigation*.[14] Drs. Goodman and Mosby found that after specific atlas adjustments, a patient who had been evaluated at the Mayo Clinic and was having ten to thirty seizures per day, had greatly reduced seizures and was able to reduce her medication by half. Dr. Young also reported on three cases of seizure disorders that responded favorably to chiropractic treatment. His findings were published in the *American Chiropractic Association Journal of Chiropractic* in 1982.[15]

These reports, as well as the study we were involved in, which we mentioned earlier, show that chiropractic can have positive effects on brain activity. Think about what a powerful statement that is: chiropractic, a treatment that is safe, with no side effects, can improve brain activity! Can you understand why we are excited about doing expanded research studies with the *StopSIDS.org* project that involve many symptoms, including those possibly related to SIDS?

Chiropractic and the Immune System

Today researchers know there is a critical link between the nerve system and the immune system. In 1974, physiologist Dr. Korr proposed that "spinal lesions" (similar to the vertebral subluxation complex) are associated with exaggerated sympathetic (a division of the nerve system) activity.[22] Sympathetic activity has been shown to release immune regulatory cells into the blood circulation, which alters immune function. This was reported by Drs. Murray, Irwin, Reardon and others.[23] The authors stated:

> *Growing evidence suggests that immune function is regulated in part by the sympathetic nervous system. Sympathetic nerve endings densely innervate lymphoid tissue such as the spleen, lymph nodes and the thymus, and lymphoid cells have beta 2 andregenergic receptors.*

In summary, the researchers were saying that the nerve system greatly affects the immune system due to the nerve supply to the critical immune system organs.

One of the most important studies showing the positive effect chiropractic care can have on the immune system and general health was performed by Ronald Pero, Ph.D., chief of cancer prevention research at New York's Preventive Medicine Institute and professor of medicine at New York University. Dr. Pero measured the immune systems of people under chiropractic care as compared to those in the general population as well as those with cancer and other serious diseases. In his initial three-year study of 107 individuals who had been under chiropractic care for five years or more, *the chiropractic patients were found to have a 200% greater immune competence than people who had not received chiropractic care, and 400% greater immune competence than people with cancer and other serious diseases.* The immune system superiority of those under chiropractic care did not diminish with age. Dr. Pero stated:

When applied in a clinical framework, I have never seen a group other than this chiropractic group to experience a 200% increase over the normal patients. This is why it is so dramatically important. We have never seen such a positive improvement in a group. . . .[24]

The chiropractic immunology connection was strengthened in 1991 when Patricia Brennan, Ph.D. and other researchers conducted a study that found improved immune response following chiropractic treatment. Specifically, the study demonstrated that phagocytic respiratory burst of polymorphnuclear neutrophils (PMN) and monocytes were enhanced in adults that had been adjusted by chiropractors .[25] In other words, the cells that act like "Pac-Man," eating and destroying bad cells are enhanced through chiropractic care.

Another important study was performed at the Sid E. Williams Research Center of Life Chiropractic College (our alma mater). The researchers took a group of HIV positive patients and adjusted their atlases over a six-month period. What they found was that the patients that were adjusted had an increase of forty-eight percent (48%) in the CD4 cells (an important immune system component). These measurements were taken at the patients' independent medical center, where they were under medical supervision for the condition. The control group (the patients that were not adjusted) did not demonstrate this dramatic increase in immune function, but actually experienced a 7.96% decrease in CD4 cell counts over the same period.[26] When we read the results of that study we were shocked that we hadn't heard about it earlier, that it didn't make the headline news or was on the front page of every newspaper. Those are very impressive results with important implications!

A paper published in 1987 found a connection between the nerve system and the immune system through endocrine channels. Dr. Felton and his team of researchers reported that the neurotransmitter norepinephrine is present in sympathetic nerve fibers that innervate lymphoid organs and act on the spleen. The authors proposed that norepinephrine in lymphoid organs plays a significant role in the regulation of the immune system. They stated:

> Stressful conditions lead to altered measures of immune function, and altered susceptibility to a variety of diseases. Many stimuli, which primarily act on the central nervous system, can profoundly alter immune responses. The two routes available to the central nervous system are neuroendocrine channels and autonomic nerve channels.[27]

Thus, the immune system can be affected by the nerve system through the connections with the endocrine and the autonomic nervous system.

In another paper published by Dr. Felton and his team, they discussed the role the nerve system plays in primary lymphoid tissue, such as bone marrow, and secondary lymphoid tissue, such as the spleen and lymph nodes. They pointed out that nerve fibers are distributed within these organs as well as along smooth muscle compartments.[28]

Another group of researchers led by Dr. Hossi described the connection between the nervous system and the immune system in 1993. The paper described how nerve cell endings in the skin, and white blood cells of the immune system, are in intimate contact. They also stated that chemicals secreted by the nerves can shut down immune system cells nearby.[29]

Dr. Udem, in his paper titled "Neural-immunologic interactions in asthma" noted that nerve stimulation can affect the growth and function of inflammatory cells.[30]

A group of researchers supported the idea that dysfunction of the nerve system can result in inflammatory syndromes, such as rheumatoid arthritis, and even behavioral syndromes such as depression. They suggested that diseases characterized by both inflammatory and emotional disturbances might begin as common alterations in specific central nervous system pathways.[31] Similar findings were reviewed by Drs. Fricchoine and Stefano as they term the connection, "neuroendocrine-neurimmune stress responses system." [32]

In another explanation of how the nerve system influences the immune system, Drs. Ottaway and Husband suggested that the nerve system plays an important role in the way lymph tissue functions. They stated:

> *Many of the alterations in the immunity resulting from CNS [central nervous system] activity may be explained in terms of changes in lymphocyte migration patterns in response to endocrine signals, neural signals via neurotransmitter release, or direct contacts between nerves and cells of the immune system.*[33]

Doctors Werhe and Krekel in their paper, "The Neoroimmune Connection in Human Tonsils," suggested the nerve system can affect the immune system by influencing vascular tone and/or permeability.[34]

Chiropractic researchers have found that fifteen minutes following a chiropractic adjustment, immune responses in the blood were significantly higher than blood collected 15 minutes before. A slight, but significant rise in substance P (another immune factor) was also noted.[35]

Dr. Christopher Kent, one of the most well respected and prolific researchers and writers in the chiropractic community, stated in his article, "Neuroimmunology and Chiropractic":

> *Contemporary research is beginning to shed light on the neurobiological mechanisms which may explain the outstanding clinical results chiropractors have been experiencing when managing patients with infectious diseases. . . . Maintaining a healthy immune system depends upon maintaining a healthy nervous system.*[36]

From these research papers it is clear to see the important role the nerve system plays on the immune system. In order to have an immune system that functions at 100%, it is important to have a spine that is functioning at 100% with no vertebral subluxations.

Medical Doctors Adjusting Infants' Atlas Vertebrae

In Germany and several other European countries it is common for medical doctors to look to the spine for improved health in infants and children. There is a specialized group of doctors that are performing similar procedures as atlas chiropractors. This specialty is called *Manual Medicine* and these doctors know that correction of the atlas area is vital to proper development and health in children.

An extremely important paper was published in 1987, in the German medical journal, *Manuelle Medizin*. Written by Dr. Gottfried Gutmann, M.D, "Blocked Atlantal Nerve Syndrome in Infants and Small Children" stressed the importance of having infants' necks (specifically the atlas) examined shortly after birth, especially if the birth is a difficult one.[11] This paper discussed the implications of the atlas blockage (atlas vertebral subluxation complex as we would call it) and the results that were gained from its correction.

In his paper, Dr. Gutmann presented three case studies from the over one thousand infants that he had treated. The infants and children were examined by palpation, observation, and x-ray analysis for the atlantal-occipital blockage (Atlas VSC). The children had symptoms that included congenital torticollis (a condition where an individual cannot straighten the neck, causing the head to be tilted towards one side) with increasing asymmetry of the face and skull, disturbed postural and muscle development, disturbed mental and especially linguistic development, recurrent tonsillitis, rhinitis, bronchitis, enteritis, and persistent conjunctivitis. Other symptoms noted were restless sleep, seizures, cerebral spasms, infantile scoliosis, and hip dysplasia. The study divided the clinical presentations into three characteristic groups of symptoms:

1. Disturbance of motor responses

2. A brain stem component

3. Children with recurrent ear, nose or throat infections.

The causes of the atlas blockage syndrome (vertebral subluxation) were attributed to birth trauma, mechanisms of delivery, and early infant or childhood trauma. Correction of the atlanto-occipital blockage was performed by specific light adjustments to the atlas vertebra. **Upon correction of the misalignment, almost without exception, all the symptoms improved**.

One of the cases Dr. Gutmann described was an eighteen-month-old boy who suffered recurring tonsillitis, frequent enteritis (an inflammation of the intestine), conjunctivitis, colds and earaches. He had extreme difficulty sleeping, refused to go to bed and would frequently wake up throughout the night screaming. His neck could not be touched due to severe pain. It was noted that this little boy had fallen several times from the diaper table as an infant. Fourteen days before his first spasm, he had fallen on the back of his head from a height of about five feet. After his first spinal adjustment the little boy slept through the night for the first time. His appetite became completely normal, and it was noted that he could walk with much more coordination than before and fell much less. As a chiropractor would say, when this child remained "in adjustment," he was asymptomatic, but following any falls or traumas, his symptoms reoccurred. Each time the symptoms returned, he was readjusted and the symptoms disappeared again.

The article went on to explain that many infants are not in autonomic balance and most of them have atlas blockages (what we call Atlas VSC). Dr. Gutmann quoted another study that examined 1,250 babies five days after birth. Of this group, 211 suffered from vomiting, hyperactivity and sleeplessness. Upon examination, 95% of these children had upper cervical strain (Atlas VSC). After being adjusted, if the strain was removed, all the infants became quiet, their muscles relaxed and the children typically fell asleep.

A study conducted by Dr. Seifert was also mentioned in Gutmann's article. Of the 1,093 newborns studied, 298 showed a correlation between atlantal-occipital blockage (Atlas VSC) and the development of a "C-scoliosis."

Dr. H. Biedermann, another German medical doctor, authored a paper titled, "Kinematic Imbalances due to Suboccipital Strain in Newborns."[37] He names a similar symptom complex to the vertebral subluxation complex, "the KISS syndrome," which has a wide range of clinical signs, and can be corrected by "manual therapy of the suboccipital segments of the upper cervical spine," what we call "an atlas adjustment." These symptoms include torticollis, c-scoliosis and motor asymmetries often associated with slowed motor development and asymmetrical hips. The risk factors include intrauterine misalignment (malposition in the womb), application of extraction aids (tools used to assist in the delivery process, such as forceps and vacuum extractor), prolonged labor and multiple fetuses (twin, triplets, etc.).

Dr. Biedermann observed that correction of the atlas area can shorten the treatment of many symptoms in infants.

Biedermann presented three case studies. One of these cases was of a six-month old girl named Charlotte. Charlotte was unable to turn her head to the left. She cried often, and her motor development was delayed. There was swelling of the right side of her face and she had a recurrent fever of unknown origin. A few hours after the first treatment, she spontaneously turned her head to the left and at her one-month check-up the swelling of her face was much less pronounced, she no longer had a fever and the motor development was improved. At a one-year check-up, no anomalies were detected.

Dr. Biedermann stated extreme cases of the KISS syndrome are "atlanto-axial rotary fixation" and are frequently diagnosed following birth injuries.

Dr. Biedermann wrote what sounds very similar to The Proprioceptive Theory we use to explain how atlas subluxations can cause abnormal brain stem function:

> *Most afferent proprioceptive signals originate from the crainiocervical junction. Any obstacle impeding these afferences will have much more extensive consequences in a nervous system in formation, which depends on appropriate stimuli to organize itself.*

He stressed the importance of proper atlas alignment, due to the fact that most of the brain development has not yet taken place in the newborn.

Dr. Biedermann stated one main reason for suboccipital strain (Atlas VSC) is due to the compromising positions that the neck and head of the infant are susceptible to during the birth process. He suggested that a majority of newborns suffer microtrauma to the brain stem. He also pointed out that there is frequent microtrauma in early childhood that can impact proper development. He stated:

> *Traumatization of the suboccipital structures inhibits functioning of the proprioceptive feedback loops. The motor development, though preprogrammed, cannot develop normally.*

In other words, because the neurological structures in the atlas area can affect normal development, when this area is compromised (through Atlas VSC), proper motor development of an infant can be disrupted. Because of the importance of the last statement, we would like you to read that again. To think of the many problems that could be prevented or improved through correcting atlas misalignments is very exciting!

As we stated earlier, Dr. Biedermann pointed out that many infants might not show any signs or symptoms but may have problems with their upper cervical spine and atlas. He mentioned a study performed by Dr. Seifert that examined a random sample of one thousand newborns and found that eleven percent (11%) had "blockages in this region." The study found of the one hundred nineteen infants with atlas blockages, seventy-eight percent (78%) showed asymmetries of the spine, such as a scoliotic posture. He stated:

> We can safely assume that most of these children would not have been considered in need of a treatment had they not been included in this study. Six percent of British primary school children have significant disorders of their visuomotor system. How many of these could profit from manual therapy of the suboccipital joints [an atlas adjustment]?

He also stated:

> These children may only show minor symptoms in the first months of their life, such as temporary fixation of the head in one position, and "recover" spontaneously. Later on—at the age of 5 or 6—they suffer headaches, postural problems or diffuse symptoms like sleep disorders, being unable to concentrate, etc.

Could this be connected to today's epidemic of A.D.D.? He stated often the problem stems from the cervical spine, and successful correction of it often proves effective. Chiropractors have also seen improvement in many attention deficit disorder children.[8, 9]

Dr. Biedermann stated that x-rays are typically necessary to determine how the correction is to be made. He also commented on the fact that some of his colleagues do not take x-rays on infants and they do not see the same positive results that he sees. He stated the treatment takes years of experience in the manual treatment of the upper cervical spine. He went on to say,

> In the hands of the experienced, the risk is minimal; we have not yet encountered any serious complications. Most children cry for a moment, but stop as soon as they are in their mother's arms. In two cases (of about 600) these children vomited after the treatment; this had no negative effect on the outcome in either case.

He went on to say that KISS (or Atlas VSC, as we would call it) is a cause of later developing scoliosis, and removal of the misalignment is the fastest and most effective way to treat the symptoms.

Dr. Biedermann noted findings similar to those that many chiropractors experience: parents will report improvement of additional symptoms after chiropractic treatment that they failed to mention at the beginning of treatment. They apparently thought there was no connection between the symptoms and the treatment, such as improved sleeping and eating habits and improved temperament.

Dr. Biedermann published another important paper with his colleagues Koch and Saternus that adds more credibility to the Atlas VSC-SIDS Theory. The paper was titled, "High Cervical Stress and Apnoea" and discussed a study that was performed at the Institute of Forensic Medicine, University of Gottingen, Germany.[38] **This study found a correlation between mechanical irritation of the suboc-**

cipital region (Atlas VSC—our term again) and infant apnea. They stated, "**. . . from this it follows that there are close relations to sudden infant death.**" This is exactly what we hope to show with the international research projects being planned through the *StopSIDS.org* Foundation.

As far back as 1921, medical doctors have been publishing papers that support chiropractic theories. When Dr. Henry Windsor published his study, little was known about the brain and nerve system in comparison to today's standards. Dr. Windsor performed autopsy studies to determine if there was a connection between minor curvatures of the spine and diseased internal organs. What he found was a nearly 100% correlation between the two. Where there was a diseased organ, a withered nerve could be traced back to the spine in most cases. His results were published in the Medical Times in 1921.[39] Dr. Windor's results stress the importance of having proper spinal alignment for overall health including the function of the internal organs.

You can see from these important studies (most from the medical profession) that an infant's atlas vertebra should be examined by a doctor of chiropractic to determine if there is any compromise to the vital nerve centers early in life. The medical literature is full of research papers that support chiropractic's theories and effectiveness. We believe an unhealthy spine can cause a number of different diseases and symptoms and that a chiropractic spinal check-up and adjustment can help in the care and prevention of sickness and disease and in the promotion of optimum health and wellness.

The Atlas Orthogonal Difference

In the chiropractic profession, there are many different effective ways of adjusting the spine to remove nerve interference. Atlas Orthogonality (pronounced or thog' ah nality) is a chiropractic program designed to find and correct spinal subluxations based on scientific and biomechanical procedures. A board-certified Atlas Orthogonist is a doctor of chiropractic that is recognized as a specialist in the field of chiropractic, with advanced training in the structure, function, and biomechanics of the upper cervical spine, specifically the atlas. The atlas vertebra is the top vertebra of the spine and because it has no bony "locks" between it and its adjacent vertebrae, as do the rest of the vertebrac in the spine, it is the most freely movable vertebra.

Most chiropractors adjust the atlas. An upper cervical or atlas chiropractor understands that the upper neck is the most important area in the spine and focuses on this area. This is not to say that upper cervical chiropractors cannot adjust other areas of the spine, or that any chiropractor cannot adjust the atlas. The atlas should be adjusted with extreme precision by a qualified chiropractor due to the critical neurological structures in this area.

Of the 60,000 chiropractors that are in practice today, there are about 1,500 that practice an upper cervical, or atlas chiropractic technique. Of that 1,500, there are only about 500 doctors that are Atlas Orthogonal (AO) chiropractors.

The Atlas Orthogonal procedure is a scientifically designed program. It is a system to reduce neurological insult by balancing anatomical structures without the use of manual manipulation. It incorporates the use of a state-of-the-art floor-based per-

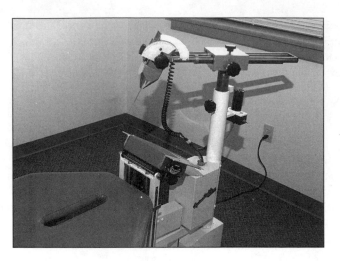

*An Atlas Orthogonal
Percussion Instrument*

cussion adjusting instrument and precision x-ray analysis. Dr. Roy Sweat of Atlanta, Georgia developed the Atlas Orthogonal procedure, including the adjusting and x-ray instruments.

Atlas Orthogonists focus on the upper neck due to the critical neurological structures located there. When the head and neck are lined up properly, the rest of the spine and nerve system work more efficiently. Shoulders and hips that have been uneven due to head tilt, often correct instantaneously when the atlas is corrected. Tight musculature in the neck also typically relaxes following an atlas correction.

The Typical Procedures in an Atlas Orthogonal Office

When a new patient arrives for care, following completion of the initial paper work, a consultation is performed. In the consultation past medical history is covered, including any symptoms the patient may be experiencing, as well as any past physical trauma. An examination will follow which typically includes a neurological, orthopedic and chiropractic examination. Included in the chiropractic examination of the

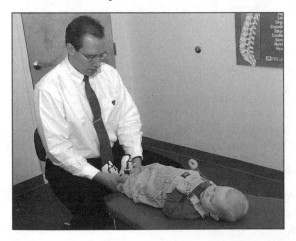

*A child having his leg length
comparison performed by Dr. Craig.*

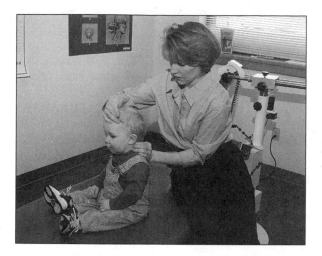

Dr. Tracey examining a child's neck by scanning palpation.

patient, two procedures are performed by the AO doctor. These are a leg-length comparison and scanning palpation of the neck. These two procedures help to determine if there is an atlas subluxation present or not.

Atlas Orthogonal Chiropractic is a gentle, safe, effective approach that does not use manipulation or cracking to correct spinal misalignments. In the Atlas Orthogonal procedure, the doctors utilize specific x-ray views of the cervical spine to see exactly how the atlas and other vertebrae have misaligned.

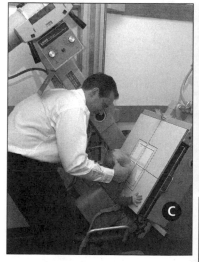

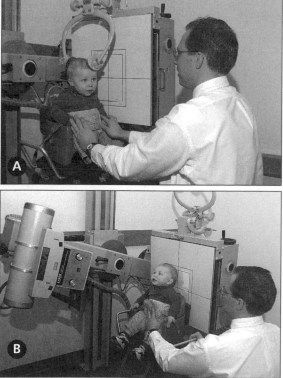

The atlas is examined in these three views, A) Sagittal, B) Frontal, and C) Horizontal to determine the three dimensional misalignment."

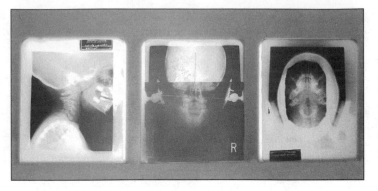

The three x-ray views that are used to determine how the atlas subluxation should be corrected. From left to right: Sagittal, frontal and horizontal.

The information received from the x-ray analysis is then used to determine the precise vectors to which the patient will be adjusted.

The Atlas Orthogonal Percussion instrument is then set with the vectors taken from the x-ray analysis, to accomplish the adjustment and correct the subluxation complex (misalignment). The patient feels no force and hears no pops or cracks. It is a painless adjustment that has proven to be one of the lightest, safest, most effective means of removing neurological insult. The AO instrument literally corrects the subluxation by introducing a percussion wave at the atlas at a predetermined angle. The instrument does not probe forward into the skin, but gently touches the patient when the adjustment is made. Most patients when adjusted with the AO instrument for the

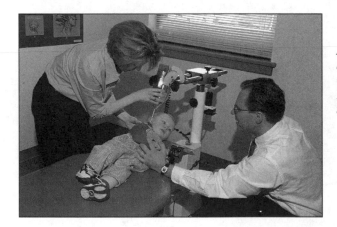

A child getting his atlas adjusted on the Atlas Orthogonal Percussion Instrument by Dr. Craig and Dr. Tracey.

first time are amazed that such a light procedure (that can hardly be felt at all) can have such dramatic effects.

Children and infants, because they have not had to go through years of misaligned and crooked spines, usually hold their adjustments longer and need fewer treatments. For a typical infant, a four-week treatment period consisting of eight to ten visits would be recommended in most cases. However, each case is treated individually and some may need more care depending on the severity of the misalignment. Periodic checkups following the initial care plan are recommended as in any other health care program.

We understand that people may have reservations about having their infant's neck x-rayed to determine how the vertebrae are misaligned. We understand that x-rays are not good for anyone, especially children, but we feel the benefits far out-weigh the risks and only take views that are necessary for the proper analysis of the atlas subluxation. A child's atlas needs to be examined carefully. It would be ineffective, and in our opinion irresponsible to guess at how an infant's neck is misaligned, because this information is too critical. Therefore, we utilize x-rays to gain the proper information needed to deliver the most effective atlas adjustment.

3

History and Update of Sudden Infant Death Syndrome

Although infants have died suddenly from unknown causes for centuries, Sudden Infant Death Syndrome (also known as "Crib Death" or "Cot Death") was first defined in 1969 as, "The sudden death of an infant or child which is unexpected by history and in which a thorough post mortem examination fails to demonstrate an adequate cause of death."[1]

The definition was then changed in 1989 to, "The sudden death of an infant under one year of age which remains unexplained after a thorough case investigation, including performance of a complete autopsy, examination of the death scene and review of the clinical history."[2] The main difference in definitions is the omission (in the second) of the statement "unexpected by history." This phrase alluded to the previously held concept that SIDS victims are completely healthy prior to death. Dr. Hannah Kinney and others stated, "This change in definition reflects perhaps the single most important lesson of SIDS research over the last 20 years, i.e. not all SIDS victims are entirely normal."[3] We suggest this lack of normal health lies in the atlas vertebral subluxation complex (Atlas VSC) and atlas neuro-vascular syndrome (ANVS). We hope to further investigate these hypotheses through international research projects that will be developed through the support of the *StopSIDS.org* Foundation.

As we mentioned in the introduction, today in the United States there are approximately 3,000 deaths each year attributed to SIDS. More children die of SIDS in one year than all children (up to age fourteen) who die of cancer, heart disease, pneumonia, child abuse, AIDS, cystic fibrosis, and muscular dystrophy combined.[4] During the past twenty-five years, over 100,000 families in the U.S. have had an infant die suddenly and unexpectedly of Sudden Infant Death Syndrome.[5]

We recognize there is some controversy in the "SIDS community" and that some investigators have suggested that every infant death be examined with suspicion. For the purpose of this book and our research, we want to approach the cause of infant death as if no inappropriate behavior has taken place.

In 1989 the number of SIDS deaths in the United States was as high as 5,634.[6] Some experts believe that the reason the number of SIDS cases has dropped dramatically in the past several years (almost 40 percent between 1992 and 1997) is due to teaching parents to put their babies to sleep on their backs or side, and not on their stomachs. We believe these results support the Atlas VSC-SIDS Theory, which is addressed more completely in Chapter Four. Briefly, we believe there is a direct relationship between the brain stem and SIDS. We know the brain stem is the control center for respiration and cardiac function. The Atlas VSC-SIDS Theory suggests that when a child has a misalignment of the atlas (the first vertebra in the neck), also called Vertebral Subluxation Complex (VSC), this causes Atlas Neuro-Vascular Syndrome (ANVS). **Associated with this syndrome is mechanical spinal cord and brain stem deformation. There may also be dysfunction of the neuro-anatomy in the brain and brain stem through the complex feedback mechanisms of the joints in the upper neck, as well as loss of normal blood supply to the brain stem through the vertebral arteries and other vascular structures in this area.** This chronic *or* acute loss of blood flow to the brain stem may cause the visible changes to the brain stem, which many researchers have identified in SIDS victims upon autopsy examination. This also may cause the brain stem to malfunction, by "short circuiting" the electrical and chemical communication between the brain and the body. This "short circuit" can cause the infant to stop breathing or his or her heart may stop and the infant may die. If a baby is put down on his or her stomach to sleep, the head must be rotated to one side so he or she can breathe. This rotation of the head can cause additional compromise to the critical neuro-anatomy and vascular supply in this area and further insult the brain stem. This brain stem insult may be increased and place an infant at greater risk of death if the infant has an atlas vertebral subluxation. With the practice of placing an infant to sleep on the back or side, a subluxated infant narrowly escapes death because there is not enough insult to the spinal cord and brain stem.

To support the idea that blood supply to the brain stem may be disrupted with neck positioning, we would like to mention one research paper here, titled "Sudden Infant Death: A Reappraisal." The authors stated,

> *Other possible death mechanisms in the prone [face down] position include . . . disruption of blood to the brain stem due to neck extension.*[7]

This disruption of blood flow to the brain stem is exactly what we have alluded to in the previous paragraph. You will see later in the book that many medical research papers have been published that address the relationship between blood supply and nerve function of the brain stem and how the two may have a direct connection with SIDS.

In his paper "Sudden Infant Death Syndrome," Dr. Dale Mortenson, a board certified Atlas Orthogonist stated,

> *I am firmly convinced that if a child has an occipital-atlanto-axial subluxation with a rotational component, which has occurred from the birth process, laying*

that child in the bed on his/her stomach, thus increasing the rotation, increases the likelihood of that child dying from S.I.D.S.[8]

We discuss other important relationships between the neck, position of the head and neck and blood supply through the vertebral arteries later in the Vertebral Artery Ischemia Theory description in the second section of Chapter Four.

The SIDS Alliance and many other groups have done a wonderful job at educating parents to put infants to sleep on their backs. However, children are still dying of SIDS. We believe one reason infants continue to succumb to SIDS, even if they are not sleeping on their stomachs, is because of abnormal brain stem function due to atlas subluxations and the Atlas Neuro-Vascular Syndrome (ANVS). These infants (that die while not on their stomachs) either have a greater degree of Atlas VSC or they have some other insult to the body that they are not able to tolerate, such as an infection, environmental or chemical stress. Regardless, we believe their condition could be improved through chiropractic treatment since research has shown this treatment is effective in increasing the body's immune function, as reported in Chapter Two.

We also believe the number of SIDS deaths has declined due to the changes in the diagnosis of the disease. In our opinion, for many years, the deaths of infants were not correctly diagnosed. Now, with increased technology and more thorough autopsies and case histories performed, the number of misdiagnosed cases has been reduced.

Despite the recent decline in the SIDS rate, Sudden Infant Death Syndrome continues to be the leading cause of death in infants between the first month and the end of the first year of life. While the various reasons and/or conditions that lead to the demise of these infants are not well understood, progress has been made in a number of areas that pertain to SIDS.[9] Approximately 60 percent of SIDS victims are boys and 40 percent girls. Infants have died from SIDS at all times of the day and night, in cribs, car seats, bassinets, and even in parents' arms. Most SIDS deaths appear to happen quietly, while the infant is sleeping. Many of the infants are found in exactly the same position in which they were put to bed. Others may have moved but there is no indication that they go through any prolonged period of pain or distress.

What Causes SIDS?

By definition, the cause of SIDS is unknown. While the exact cause and mechanism of death is not yet known, we do know that SIDS is not contagious.[9]

No obvious or consistent warning signs occur that might alert us to the risk of SIDS. Sometimes the infant was not feeding quite so well on the day he or she died, or there may have been symptoms of a slight cold or stomach upset. It seems that while minor infections of some sort or another are frequently found in SIDS babies, on careful post-mortem examination, these infections are mild and seem in themselves to be an inadequate cause of sudden death.[9] However, here again we must mention that VSC can lower the body's resistance to infection and disease and even these minor illnesses, when combined with VSC and ANVS, may be too much for an infant to overcome.

Many research papers have debated the question of "at-risk infants." Meaning, are there any signs, symptoms or characteristics that may determine that an infant is at an increased risk of SIDS? There have been credible arguments on both sides. Some say there are signs and symptoms that we can recognize and to which we should give extra attention. These include sleep apnea, an apparent life threatening episode (ALTE), increased heart rate, extremely premature infants, those with moderate to severe broncho-pulmonary problems, neurological disorders, abnormal brain stem function and certain disorders or diseases that the mother may have had during pregnancy. Other researchers feel there are no factors that can warn that an infant may die of SIDS. This lack of distinct warning signs makes it difficult to do any research on effective treatment methods that may help to prevent SIDS. We believe that if an infant had an ALTE, where he or she stopped breathing, possibly turned blue and had to be resuscitated, this infant would have been diagnosed as SIDS, had there been no intervention.

One of the first research projects that will be performed through *StopSIDS.org* will involve infants that have had an ALTE or that have any type of apnea (which means they stop breathing) or any respiratory dysfunction, such as infant asthma. We will let the "experts" debate whether or not these infants could have become SIDS victims. If we can show that through chiropractic atlas adjusting, these episodes and symptoms are reduced, this will be a tremendous contribution to infant health.

Dr. Ronald Harper, and his research team from UCLA, in collaboration with scientists at the Brompton Hospital and the University of Sheffield in Great Britain, made incredible strides in identifying subtle risk factors in infants who later died of SIDS. These researchers recorded heart and breathing patterns in 6,914 apparently normal, healthy infants that ranged in age from two to 65 days. Sixteen of the infants in this group later died of SIDS. The investigators then compared the physiologic recordings (detailed health functions) of the 16 SIDS victims to 35 recordings of age-matched control infants.[10]

Unlike previous studies that used gross measures of respiratory rate, and found no differences in overall respiratory rate or variation, this study used a unique measure, originally designed to detect changes in heart rate, to plot the amount of time from one breath to the next, or the breath-to-breath interval. Using this approach, the investigators were able to compare each breath-to-breath interval to the previous one while controlling for breathing rate. They found that infants who later died of SIDS exhibited less variation in breath-to-breath intervals at slow breathing rates during sleep than did infants who survived. Specifically, breaths following long breaths showed less change in infants who later died. This finding indicates a more "rigid" control of respiration, and, theoretically, less responsiveness to physiologic input than that found in the control infants. "If you look at the moment-to-moment changes, what you find is that at very slow breathing rates, such as those found during sleep, infants that later die don't change their breathing intervals as much as normal infants," said project investigator Dr. Harper. He also stated in the paper:

> *The altered breathing patterns suggest a subtle difference in the control of breathing in infants who die of SIDS.* **Such a difference points to the brain** *areas which fail when vulnerable infants encounter a potentially lethal* **respiratory challenge during sleep.**

We believe this statement offers more support of the Atlas VSC-SIDS Theory which says an atlas subluxation can adversely affect the brain stem, which in turn, affects breathing.

Most researchers agree that a large percentage of SIDS victims have something in common. This finding is an oxygen deprivation called hypoxia. It is believed that this hypoxia causes the changes found during autopsies in the liver, brown fat and areas of the brain stem. These findings support the Atlas VSC-SIDS Theory, and in our opinion, provide visual proof of a condition that was caused by an Atlas VSC and ANVS, which contributes to SIDS. Again, we will get into much greater detail in Chapter Four, but briefly, when the atlas is misaligned at least three things can take place:

1. Minor spinal cord and brainstem distortion

2. The electrical and chemical signals to and from the brain get "confused"

3. Blood supply to the brain stem and other critical areas of the brain may be decreased through vertebral artery ischemia (lack of blood) and venous blood pooling, resulting in hypoxia (a decrease in oxygen).

Vaccines as a Cause of SIDS

For years many people have questioned whether certain vaccinations given to newborns could be a cause of SIDS in some babies. Although there are medical authorities who deny any correlation, we asked The National Sudden Infant Death Syndrome Resource Center for references to a Vaccination-SIDS link. They were extremely helpful and provided us with 70 abstracts from research papers published in scientific journals that discuss this topic.

Because it is such a highly controversial issue, we do not want to distract focus from the Atlas VSC-SIDS Theory or make any statements on whether or not vaccinations have been a contributing factor to SIDS. We would however encourage every individual who is faced with the difficult decision of whether or not to vaccinate a child, to become informed on all the benefits and risks. There are many excellent books available on the subject and with today's computer technology, one can also access the Internet for a wide range of information. One can obtain information from the National Vaccine Information Center, in Vienna, Virginia. The Web site address is www.909shot.com.

The United States infant mortality rate is too high

We have made incredible strides and improvements in the health and medical field, including obstetrics and gynecology. In the United States, we have access to the greatest, high-tech treatment procedures in the world. For instance, today a defect in a fetal heart can be recognized and corrected prior to or shortly after birth. Why then is the United States twenty-third when it comes to the infant mortality rate? In other words, why does an infant have a better chance of surviving in twenty-three other countries than in the United States? We believe this is due to the mentality that has been around in the U.S. for so long. This mentality is one of a "quick fix," of "treat the symptoms" and get rid of pain. For too long, we have not looked at the root of the problem, but have played patch medical care. Along with the popularity of alternative and complementary medicine, we hope this book serves as a logical approach to true "prevention" and wellness care through atlas chiropractic maintenance starting in infancy and continuing on throughout life.

4

Correcting Vertebral Misalignments and the Atlas VSC-SIDS Theory

We are not the first to suggest Sudden Infant Death Syndrome (SIDS) has a possible link to the upper cervical spine. Dr. Palmer associated cervical spinal cord injury with fetal death in 1910,[1] as did Dr. Crothers in 1923[2] and Dr. Gilles in 1979.[3] More recently, numerous medical and chiropractic researchers have suggested the relationship between SIDS and the brain stem, spinal cord and/or upper cervical spine.[4-16] In fact there are well over 100 scientific research papers that point to the brain stem as a critical link to SIDS. In this chapter we want to show how the Atlas Vertebral Subluxation Complex (VSC) and the Atlas Neuro-Vascular Syndrome (ANVS) may explain the cause of a large percentage of SIDS cases.[17] Again, we call this connection The Atlas VSC-SIDS Theory. Further, we also want to offer a possible solution to this tragedy.

Due to the fact that there is a lot of information to discuss regarding the spine, and how chiropractic may play a preventative role in SIDS, we have divided this chapter into two sections. Section One is designed for the general public. Section Two is designed for the person who has more medical knowledge and who understands more technical terms. We give detailed examples of the medical research that has been reported to date establishing the fact that brain stem malfunction is possibly the main reason infants succumb to SIDS. We realize many parents will want to ask their pediatricians what they think about this theory, therefore Section Two is more detailed.

SECTION I
The Atlas VSC-SIDS Theory

As stated earlier, unless one has a crystal ball and can see into the future, there is no way that SIDS prevention can be proven, since it is only evident and diagnosed after the fact (of death). For this reason, we have chosen to focus our research studies on symptoms that are related to SIDS, such as breathing and brain stem abnormalities, and other infant related disorders. We believe that once we have established that adjusting the atlas vertebra can help infants with these symptoms, the next logical step will be to have all infants checked for atlas subluxations shortly after birth. We believe the only way to see another major decrease in the rate of SIDS is to have every infant examined by a chiropractor and when necessary, have his or her atlas adjusted to remove the subluxation.

The Atlas VSC-SIDS Theory is defined as,

A theory that incorporates the relationship between the first bone in the spine (C-1, also known as the atlas) and the critical neurological and vascular structures that affect cardiac and respiratory function, that are located in this area, as a cause of SIDS. This theory recognizes that there may be other causes of SIDS, and this is presented as one theory.

When an atlas (the first vertebra in the spine) becomes subluxated in an infant the following can take place:

- *Abnormal spinal cord and brain stem function due to direct mechanical stretching of these structures.*
- *Electrical and chemical signals to and from the brain become disturbed.*
- *A decrease in the proper blood supply to the brain stem from the vertebral arteries which may be altered due to the malposition of the atlas.*

Due to the fact that the infant nerve system and brain stem are not fully matured, infants are at particular risk of serious health consequences from nerve system insult.

Summary of Related SIDS Research

The fact that vertebrae can be subluxated to the point of decreasing normal nerve transmission has been well established. So the question to be answered is, "Can a subluxation cause SIDS?" We believe the evidence strongly suggests it can.

One important development in the focus on brain stem research and how it relates to SIDS took place in 1992, when the SIDS Alliance established the first Center of Excellence for Brainstem Research for SIDS at the Pediatric Neuroscience Center at Boston Children's Hospital and Harvard University under the coordination of Dr. Hannah Kinney. Utilizing experts from the Departments of Neurology, Neurosurgery and Pathology, Dr. Kinney has been able to conduct a series of integrated studies of the brain and brain stem of infants. These multidisciplinary studies have also received funding from the National Institute of Child Health and Human Development (NICHHD).

Dr. Kinney and her colleagues are testing the idea that SIDS, or a subset of SIDS, is due to a developmental brain stem defect in autonomic and/or respiratory control during sleep. Focusing specifically on the arcuate nucleus in the ventral medulla area of the brain stem, which is important in the detection of carbon dioxide and other respiratory and blood pressure responses, this team is identifying abnormalities that put an infant at risk for sudden death during sleep. While continuing to study the anatomy and neurochemistry of the ventral medulla in SIDS victims, Dr. Kinney's team is also looking at the function and pathology of the ventral medulla in animal models. The ultimate goals of this research are to define ventral medullary abnormalities in living infants, and to define ways of preventing the abnormalities from leading to sudden infant death.

We believe that correction of atlas subluxations may be an effective method of removing brain stem insult, thus preventing SIDS. We hope through research efforts, it will be demonstrated that these beliefs are correct.

As we mentioned earlier, a team of researchers at UCLA, led by Dr. Ronald Harper, has also performed vital research that represents hope that SIDS may be prevented by early intervention. Dr. Harper and his team identified a breathing abnormality in SIDS victims. The researchers said, "The findings from this new study offer the hope of eventually developing screening tests to identify infants who are at risk."[18] **We are anticipating that chiropractic examination of the upper cervical spine will be that screening test.**

Other studies by Dr. Harper, his colleagues and other researchers have identified abnormal heart-rate variability in infants who later died of SIDS.[19–23] We believe these findings are consistent with the brain stem being compromised by subluxations at the atlas area. Other researchers have identified subtle sleep characteristics associated with a higher risk of SIDS which we also believe may be caused by an atlas subluxation.[24–38]

How the Upper Cervical Spine Can Affect the Spinal Cord and Brain Stem

There are numerous explanations as to how an upper cervical subluxation can affect the central nervous system including the brain stem.[39–48] Neuroscience is proving that structural integrity, particularly the structural integrity of the upper cervical spine, with its various intimate relationships with several neural components, has a direct influence on the nervous system's assessment and coordination of whole body function, mainly health. An atlas subluxation complex and the atlas neuro-vascular syndrome (ANVS) may cause neurological and vascular compromise to the spinal cord and brain stem. We would like to focus on three different mechanisms that may cause spinal cord and brain stem dysfunction, and ultimately SIDS. By no means do we present these as being the only relationships that may cause the necessary neurological involvement, but we believe these explanations are scientifically sound and accepted:

1. The Dentate Ligament Cord Distortion Hypothesis
2. The Proprioceptive Insult Hypothesis

3. The Vertebral Artery Ischemia Theory.

In this section we will briefly explain these three mechanisms and how they each affect the normal function of the brain stem. In Section II, we give detailed explanations of these theories and mechanisms.

1. THE DENTATE LIGAMENT CORD DISTORTION HYPOTHESIS

This theory suggests that an upper cervical misalignment (at the occipital-atlanto-axial area, C-0, C-1 and C-2), due to the attachments of the ligaments in this area, can actually cause *direct* mechanical irritation to the upper spinal cord and brain stem. This theory also suggests that the blood flow in this area can be altered by an upper cervical subluxation due to the fact that these vascular structures are more vulnerable than other areas of the body, and can be impaired by dentate ligament distortion.

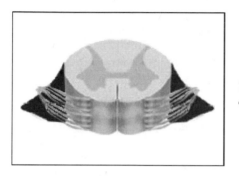

The spinal cord in the upper cervical spine demonstrating the dentate ligament connections.

Dentate ligament distortion has proven to have far reaching effects on the nerve system. Upper cervical cord lesions were found to have a profound degenerative effect on the nervous system.[49]

In 1967 dentate ligament distortion was found to be related to kinking of the brain stem (specifically the medulla oblongata) in children.[50]

2. THE PROPRIOCEPTIVE INSULT HYPOTHESIS

This theory focuses on the unique anatomy of the joints of the upper cervical verte-brae to explain how a VSC in this area can interfere with normal brain stem function. In the joint capsules, receptors feed information back to the brain through a series of connections (called synapses). These receptors in the joints are called *mechano-receptors*, and are the largest sensory axons in the body. The *upper neck* is the area in the body with the most mechanoreceptors. When these joints lose their proper position, range of motion, or become subluxated, the mechanoreceptors do not work properly and the information that is supposed to go to and from the brain may get distorted.

It has been shown that 50% of the neurons in the brain are driven by mechanorecep-tors; therefore, their role is critical and it is extremely important that they function properly. When a dysfunctional joint causes a mechanoreceptor to send distorted messages to the brain, the brain cannot interpret the information correctly and may send improper signals back through the nervous system, including the autonomic nerve system, which controls cardiac function and respiration. These signals sent from the brain may adversely affect our health.

A chiropractic adjustment is designed to restore a vertebra to its proper position and improve its range of motion back to its normal level. The goal of an atlas adjustment is to correct the relationship between the occiput (the skull) and the first two vertebrae: the atlas (C1) and the axis (C-2). When this is accomplished, the mechanoreceptors in the joints are once again able to transmit the necessary information to and from the brain accurately, carrying out the necessary functions, and sending the proper signals to coordinate health in the body.

3. THE VERTEBRAL ARTERY ISCHEMIA THEORY

The vertebral arteries, which supply blood to the brain stem and other critical brain centers, come up to the brain through small openings in the neck vertebrae of C6 through C1 on both sides. These openings are called vertebral transversarii. Excessive amounts of rotation and extension in the upper neck can cause compromise to the vertebral arteries, leading to lack of proper blood supply, thus decreasing oxygen-

A drawing of the upper neck from the front and from the side showing the vertebral arteries as they enter the head.

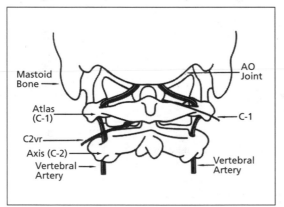

FIGURE A.

AO Joint is the Atlanto-Occipital Joint, Pointing to C1 is the C-1 Nerve Root, C2VR is the C2 Ventral Rami.

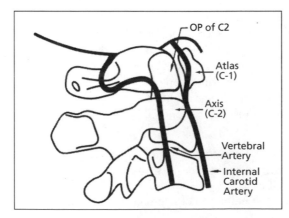

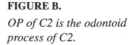

FIGURE B.

OP of C2 is the odontoid process of C2.

ation of the area being supplied. In Section Two of this chapter, we will cite numerous research projects that have demonstrated this. We believe that with the atlas neurovascular syndrome, the nerves in this area can also cause abnormal blood flow through the vertebral arteries when they are irritated.

During many births, the physician or attendant will rotate the infant's head to help the delivery process. This head rotation may be the first cause of Atlas VSC and atlas neuro-vascular syndrome, and the first step in the malfunctioning of the brain stem and vagus nerve.

The vagus nerve, which affects many vital life processes such as breathing, heart rate, blood flow and control of the internal organs, has its nuclei (or origin) in the brain stem. Therefore, if there is vertebral artery ischemia, the vagus nerve can be adversely affected, thus disturbing normal respiration, cardiac function and other autonomic responses.

In an article published in 1995, Dr. D.W. Walker demonstrated that low blood oxygen levels in newborn and fetal sheep caused breathing to stop. The article stated that the exact mechanism behind this is unknown, but offered a possible reason that pointed to the brain stem.[51] We believe an atlas subluxation in an infant can cause the vertebral arteries, which supply the blood to the brain stem, to malfunction. This results in an inadequate supply of oxygen for the normal function of the brain stem and breathing stops.

With this information, we believe that an atlas subluxation involving the occiput, atlas and axis can compromise the function of the vertebral arteries. This compromise can cause ischemia and malfunction of the brain stem and the vagus nerve. Involvement of these critical structures can compromise an infant's health and respiratory function, and ultimately lead to death.

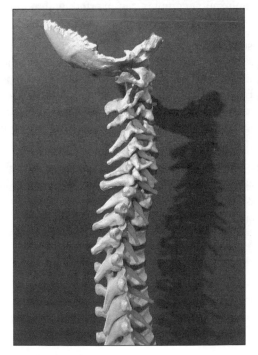

A model of the spine that shows the vertebral arteries as they travel up the cervical spine.

Along with these three theories of how an atlas subluxation can affect the brain stem and cause SIDS, we would like to mention one other theory that has been in the chiropractic profession for many years that may explain a spine-nerve system-chiropractic-SIDS relationship. This theory is the Neuorodystrophic Hypothesis, which states that when the nervous system is irritated through VSC, the body may suffer in several predictable ways. One of the most significant effects is a partial shutdown of the immune system with resulting lowered resistance to disease. Recent research has shown very involved connections between the nervous system and the immune system, even producing evidence that nerve fibers go to almost every lymphocyte in a lymph node. With this hypothesis, we can better understand why an infant with an Atlas VSC could succumb to SIDS while suffering from an otherwise mild childhood disease or infection, and how adjusting an infant (correcting its Atlas VSC) has great ramifications on the long-term health of that individual.

The Neuorodystrophic Hypothesis also helps to explain why children who have been sick with various childhood maladies and diseases, such as asthma, allergies and ear infections, get well under chiropractic care. It also helps to explain why, despite exposure to sick children from day care through first grade, our own three children, ages seven, five and one, have never been on an antibiotic in their lives. We are not saying they are never sick or catch a cold, but they have never needed any drugs. Their bodies have a tremendous ability to heal themselves very quickly.

Medical Research Supporting the Atlas VSC-SIDS Theory

Today's knowledge of human neuroanatomy and physiology and the three theories of how an Atlas VSC can adversely affect the brain stem, allow us to explain how an occipito-atlanto-axial subluxation complex can interfere with normal brain stem function.

The notion that vertebral subluxation may contribute to nervous system dysfunction is corroborated by the German medical doctor, Gottfried Gutmann, whom we mentioned earlier. He wrote one of the strongest papers ever written that supports children getting their atlas checked and adjusted by a chiropractor.[52] He stated that over 1,000 children were treated successfully (almost without exception) for a variety of ailments, by spinal adjustments at the atlas. Symptoms reported to have responded favorably include:

- congenital torticollis (a condition where an individual cannot straighten the neck, causing the head to be tilted towards one side) with increasing asymmetry of the face and skull
- disturbed mental and especially linguistic development
- recurrent rhinitis
- bronchitis
- tonsillitis
- enteritis (inflammation of the intestine)
- persistent conjunctivitis

- restless sleep with crying out at night
- unmotivated central seizures
- cerebral spasms
- disturbed motor responses with frequent falls
- infantile scoliosis
- distortion of the iliosacral joint
- so-called "growing pains"
- disturbance of the appetite
- overall inability to thrive

Gutmann mentioned a study by Lewit who found that among primarily youthful patients with chronic tonsillitis, 92% had an atlanto-occipital joint blockage, primarily between the occiput and the atlas. He remarked, "If the indications are correctly observed, chiropractic can often bring about amazingly successful results, because the therapy is a causal one." [52] Dr. Gutmann also mentioned that a colleague of his, named Dr. Mohn, had reported to him that when the atlas disturbance was corrected in children, no tonsillectomy was needed.

Dr. Gutmann stated,

> *Surveillance of infants should involve the observations of motor development and manual control of the a-o (atlanto-occipital) joints. This should be obligatory in difficult births especially with congenital torticollis. With developmental disturbances of every kind, the atlanto-occipital joints should be examined and in each case be treated manually in a qualified manner.* **The success of this treatment eclipses every other attempt at treatment, including especially the use of medications.** [52]

Isn't it frustrating that although a German medical doctor suggested in 1952 that there is a connection between the upper neck and brain stem function in children, American patients continue to be questioned and harassed by their medical doctor when they discuss wanting to bring their children to a chiropractor?

It is clear that an upper cervical misalignment can adversely affect critical nervous system anatomy and physiology. Therefore, we hope the Atlas VSC-SIDS Theory gets the attention it deserves in the scientific community, as well as by the general public. Although it is sure to meet a considerable amount of resistance, we agree with Dr. Smith, a medical doctor who suggested that every newborn be given a spinal examination with particular attention given to the upper cervical spine.[53] This examination should be done by a chiropractor, and if subluxations are found, an adjustment should be given.

What Medical Doctors Say about Atlas Orthogonality

Recall from Chapter Two that Atlas Orthogonality is a type of chiropractic which focuses on adjusting the atlas vertebra (the top vertebra of the spine, located just beneath the brain stem) with a special percussion adjusting instrument. Here are some comments demonstrating support for this type of chiropractic, as well as chiropractic in general, from members of the medical profession:

- *The Atlas Orthogonal Program is a great asset to the health care field and should be incorporated into the main stream medical approach towards good health. It is also my opinion that the Atlas Orthogonal Program should be a specialty field in chiropractic, like orthopedics is a specialty in the medical field.*

  Having access to the Atlas Orthogonal work has been a tremendous additional instrument in helping our patients.

  On a personal note, I have been adjusted by Dr. Robert Kornek and Dr. Beverly Martin with excellent results for migraines and cervical radiculitis.

  DR. CRAIG UNDERSET, M.D., LaGrange, Georgia

- *I have referred many patients with cervical spine problems to Dr. Roy Sweat [the developer of the atlas orthogonal adjusting procedure] over the years, and have been very satisfied with the help that he has given to them. I believe the Atlas Orthogonal work is a very valuable tool that, used correctly, could help many, many people.*

  DR. NICHOLAS GONZALES, MD, Immunologist, Cancer Specialist

- *I have been very satisfied with the results I have received through Atlas Orthogonal Chiropractic from Dr. Craig Wehrenberg. Both my wife and I have seen significant improvement in a relatively short period of time. One of the things I like most is the safety of the procedure, with no side effects.*

  DR. RICHARD SULKOW, Anesthesiologist, Troy, New York

- *I have seen unbelievable physiological improvement with Atlas Orthogonal Chiropractic. This is the type of work that is going on out there that the medical profession does not know is going on, and they have to be made aware of it.*

  DR. COULTER RULE, MD, Internal Medicine, Psychiatrist and Retired New York State Medical Board Examiner

- *For many families in the United States, chiropractic care is no longer an alternative, but an integral part of regular health care, both for health promotion and the treatment of common diseases.*

  ANNE CC LEE, BSE; DAWN H. LI, MD; KATHI J. KEMPER, MD, MPH in their article, "Chiropractic Care for Children" published in *The Archives of Pediatric and Adolescent Medicine*, April 2000;Vol. 154, No. 4: pages 401–407.

- *We've been able to put together a scientific explanation of how neck structure causes headaches . . . not all headaches, but a significant number of them. Chiropractors have been saying that for years. Unfortunately, many (medical) doctors tend to have a jaundiced view of chiropractors but they (chiropractors) were right about headaches.*

  PETER ROTHBART, M.D., IRCPC President of the North America Cervicogenic Headache Society

- *I am astonished with the help I have gotten with Atlas Orthogonal Chiro-practic.*

DR. BETTY GESSEL, MD

- *In a three-year study of 107 individuals who had been under chiropractic care for five years or more, the chiropractic patients were found to have a 200% greater immune competence than people who had not received chiro-practic care, and a 400% greater immune competence than people with cancer and other serious diseases.*

R. PERO, PH.D.
Chief of Cancer Prevention Research at New York's Preventive Medicine Institute, 1989

SIDS Screening Methods Need to be Developed

Since there have not been any standard screening procedures established to identify an infant that might be at risk of SIDS, *we suggest every child be screened for subluxations of the atlas area by a chiropractor shortly after birth*. Chiropractic is the most efficient method of finding and removing life threatening and health compromising nerve interference.

Two former chiropractic interns agreed with this suggestion in their paper titled "The Interface between Sudden Infant Death Syndrome and Chiropractic."[54] The authors, Andrew Bonci and Conrad Wynne conclude:

> *It would certainly be within the scope of the chiropractic profession to devise a protocol for the screening of SIDS candidates, to monitor their neuromusculo-skeletal development and maintain the proper integrity of the cervical spine. Chiropractic may be able to reestablish the integrity of the cervical spine. By doing so, vertebrobasilar perfusion will improve, neuronal tension and com-promise can be alleviated and maturational lag in the central nervous system can be equilibrated.*

As we mentioned earlier, our belief that all infants should have their necks ex-amined is further supported by the fact that in 1989 the National Institute of Child Health and Human Development convened an expert panel to review SIDS, which developed the following, revised definition for SIDS: "The sudden death of an infant under one year of age which remains unexplained after a thorough case inves-tigation, including performance of a complete autopsy, examination of the death scene and review of the clinical history."[55] A critical difference between this defini-tion and the previous description used in SIDS research, which was set forth in 1969,[56] is the omission of the statement "unexpected by history." This phrase alluded to the previously held concept that SIDS victims were completely healthy prior to death. Dr. Kinney and others stated, "This change in definition reflects perhaps the single most important lesson of SIDS research over the last 20 years, i.e. not all SIDS victims are entirely normal."[4] We suggest this lack of normal health lies in the occipito-atlanto-axial subluxation complex and the Atlas Neuro-Vascular Syndrome, which can cause abnormal respiration functions and other health problems. We plan to further investigate these hypotheses through research performed in conjunction with the *StopSIDS.org* Foundation.

In their paper "Sudden Infant Death Syndrome and Chiropractic," Drs. Kent and Gentempo stated:

> *Every seasoned chiropractor who has adjusted infants knows the dramatic responses which often follow the correction of a subluxation. Chiropractic care for newborns is immensely rich in clinical promise. Besides the possible link between subluxation and SIDS, the lifelong health benefits, which may follow adjustment shortly after birth, should be the subject of additional research. As chiropractors, we have a public health responsibility to further explore the relationship between SIDS and subluxation.*[7]

As chiropractors have stated for years, the steps a sick individual should take to regain health should be:

1. Chiropractic

2. Drugs with side effects

3. Irreversible surgery

Too often the chiropractor is the last resort that a sick person tries, but the results achieved are far better than the previous treatments. We propose that parents consider aiming the life of a newborn towards good health by *beginning* with chiropractic, and pursuing medical treatment as necessary after that.

SECTION II
Atlas VSC-SIDS Theory: Advanced Medical Explanation

WARNING: *In this section we cover scientific research with a lot of medical terms. We have included technical information so that the general public can show this to pediatricians if they want their opinion on chiropractic atlas care for their children.*

Brief Anatomy and Physiology Review

Respiration, cardiac function and other critical autonomic functions are under direct control of the brain stem.[57] The respiratory center is composed of several widely dispersed groups of neurons located on both sides of the medulla oblongata and pons. It is divided into three major collections of neurons:

1. A dorsal respiratory group, located in the dorsal (back) portion of the medulla which mainly causes inspiration (breathing in).

2. A ventral (front) respiratory group located in the ventrolateral (front and side) part of the medulla, which can cause either expiration (breathing out) or inspiration, depending upon which neurons in the group are stimulated.

3. The pneumotaxic center, located dorsally (back) in the superior (upper)

portion of the pons which helps control both the rate and pattern of breathing. The dorsal respiratory group of neurons plays the fundamental role in the control of respiration.

Dr. Towbin stated, "Life for the newborn depends, not on the forebrain, but on the preservation and the healthy function of the brainstem and upper spinal cord, that section of the central nervous system which holds the respiratory and other vital centers."[58]

To impress upon the reader the importance the brain stem has on SIDS, we want to provide you with some of the most relevant medical research papers that have been published on the subject. This selection is only a fraction of more than 100 articles written on the brain stem-SIDS relationship. We understand that for the majority of readers, much of the terminology used may be hard to understand, but those who have studied this syndrome or have a knowledge of anatomy will appreciate much of the following.

This first paper does everything but state our theory. In **"The Interest of the Neurological Tissue Preservation for the Investigation of Sudden Infant Death Syndrome"**[59] Lucena and Cruz-Sanchez stated:

> *Brain stem dysfunction of circuits that control respiration and cardiovascular stability may be involved in SIDS. It is postulated that this abnormality originates in utero and leads to sudden death during a vulnerable postnatal period.*

This supports the Atlas VSC-SIDS Theory, which suggests atlas subluxations can occur in utero. We want to emphasize that an atlas VSC may also be the result of trauma during the birth process, or an event early in the infant's life that causes the spine to be misplaced. We believe it is an atlas subluxation which causes the nerve circuits to malfunction and leads to abnormal brain stem function, resulting in SIDS.

In their paper **"Abnormal Brainstem Auditory Evoked Potentials in Infants with Threatened Sudden Infant Death Syndrome,"**[60] Orlowski and others described the results of brain stem auditory evoked potentials on ten infants who were classified as "at risk for SIDS." A brain stem auditory evoked potential (BAEP) is a physiological examination to test the function of the brain stem. All ten of the infants tested were found to have abnormal BAEP tests. These findings were compared to normal BAEP tests in two infants with apnea (a problem in which an infant stops breathing) secondary to mechanical airway obstruction, in two infants with cyanotic congenital heart disease, and six normal control infants. They said,

> *BAEP tests should prove useful in prospectively studying infants with life threatening apnea, evaluating therapeutic modalities, and possibly as a screening tool to identify infants at risk. **The abnormal BAEP implicates the respiratory center and brainstem as the area of dysfunction in SIDS.***

In other words, if the child had a "near miss for SIDS" incident and did not have an obstruction to their airway or some congenital problem with their respiratory center, the problem was found to be in their brain stem. This is *critical* information! Our plans at *StopSIDS.org* are to perform BAEP tests prior to and following adjustment, to determine if atlas adjusting can have positive effects on this test.

In their article **"Obstructive Sleep Apnea and Near-Miss for SIDS: I. Report of an**

Infant with Sudden Death,[61] Guilleminault and others reported on an infant girl who died of SIDS. This child, when compared with other control and near-miss infants, had the highest number of apneic events; she also had increased heart rate during some of the apneic events. Upon autopsy, a complete gross and microscopic examination showed no pathological changes except for **"a fibrillary gliosis in the raphe nuclei of the pons and medulla."** Fibrillary gliosis is an excessive accumulation of "nerve helper/repair cells" that come to a site after some type of damage or injury has taken place. In our opinion this gliosis was secondary to an Atlas VSC and the ANVS, which caused chronic hypoxia in this area of the brain stem. The authors stated, "More intensive studies of the midline structures of the brain stem in SIDS infants dying of unknown causes are also recommended."

In the paper titled, **"The Interrelationship between Sudden Infant Death Syndrome and Sleep Apnea Syndrome,"** Lemmi and others noted a relationship of abnormal BAEP tests in both infants and adults with sleep apnea.[62]. This finding suggests a problem with brain stem function that we believe can be caused by an Atlas VSC and can be improved upon by atlas adjusting.

In **"The Brain Stem in Sudden Infant Death Syndrome: A Postmortem Survey,"** Summers and Parker stated, "Abnormal central neural regulation of respiration may be involved in the pathogenesis [cause] of SIDS." They found medullary gliosis in the reticular formation in 12% of the 34 SIDS victims studied. The reticular formation plays a critical role in respiratory and cardiovascular control. The authors stated: "These findings support the need for more extensive prospective neuropathological investigations in SIDS utilizing more sophisticated techniques."[63]

Schulte and others in **"Neuronal Control of Neonatal Respiration—Sleep Apnea and the Sudden Infant Death Syndrome"** stated, "Brain mechanisms may be responsible for both sleep apnea and serious apneic events. These mechanisms may involve immature respiratory neurons, faulty chemoreceptor or mechanoreceptor regulation of breathing, or weak intercostal muscle strength reflexes."[64] We believe all of these may be a result of the Atlas VSC and ANVS. They also pointed out that severe apneic episodes, which may be termed "near-miss-for-SIDS," do occur in the same population as SIDS and are related to similar risk factors.

Another paper that shows support for the brain stem-SIDS connection, was written by Dr. Atkinson and others. In **"Ischemia of the Brain Stem as a Cause of Sudden Infant Death Syndrome"** the authors stated:

> *Recent evidence indicates that the sudden infant death syndrome (SIDS) is related to abnormal control of respiration. Focal morphologic changes have not been noted. In a case of SIDS, ischemic degeneration was noted bilaterally in the medulla, particularly in the dorsal motor nucleus of the vagus nerve. Pathologic changes were not found elsewhere in the CNS. To our knowledge, this is the first description of a focal brain-stem lesion in SIDS that had enough of a role in altered respiratory control to cause death.*[65]

This paper is important because it found effects of vascular changes in the brain stem, specifically at the vagus nerve. We believe the Atlas VSC can cause the vertebral arteries (which supply the blood to this area) to be compromised. Therefore we theorize that the Atlas VSC can cause brain stem malfunction through vertebral artery compromise.

In "**Reactive Gliosis in the Medulla Oblongata of Victims of the Sudden Infant Death Syndrome**," Dr. Kinney and others found that their study reinforced previous observations that an abnormality of the brain stem occurred in a group of SIDS victims in contrast to a group of control infants.[66]

In their paper "**Possible Role of the Brain Stem in Sudden Infant Death Syndrome**" Baba and others discussed how defects in the central respiratory control can cause SIDS. They discussed that brain stem dendrite changes may have a role in SIDS and suggest more research needs to be performed in order to provide a more definitive answer on this relationship.[67]

Dr. Naeye, in the paper "**Brain-Stem and Adrenal Abnormalities in the Sudden Infant Death Syndrome**," found 14 of 28 SIDS victims had abnormal findings in their brain stems as well as in their adrenal medullas. They believed these findings were due to chronic hypoxemia. We believe this chronic hypoxemia is a result of the vertebral subluxation complex and of ANVS, as it can affect the flow of blood through the vertebral arteries.[68]

"**Brainstem Dysfunction in the Infant Apnea Syndrome**" by Orlowski and others is strong evidence for the brain stem-SIDS relationship.[69] In this paper, the researchers studied thirty-six infants identified as having infant apnea syndrome (IAS) and twenty-five control infants with a comparable age distribution. These infants were evaluated with Brainstem Auditory Evoked Potential (BAEP) testing. Fifteen IAS patients had bilateral abnormalities (problems on both sides), and twenty-one IAS patients had unilateral abnormalities (abnormalities on one side). In other words, ***all the infants with Infant Apnea Syndrome had an abnormal BAEP***, which suggests the apnea may have been caused by an abnormally functioning brain stem.

In their paper "**Brainstem Auditory Evoked Responses in Infants at Risk of Sudden Infant Death**," Pettigrew and Rahilly found that a significant number of infants who were at risk for SIDS had an abnormal BAEP as compared to a control group.[70] The authors suggest that "maturation of neural processing in the brainstem of these infants may be delayed." We believe this delay in maturation of neural processing is due to the Atlas Vertebral Subluxation Complex and the atlas neuro-vascular syndrome, as we believe the Atlas VSC can cause decreased blood supply, which may lead to a lack of development at this critical neurological structure.

The paper "**Brainstem Immaturity in Sudden Infant Death Syndrome: A Quantitative Rapid Golgi Study of Dendritic Spines in 95 Infants**," the authors Quattrochi and others studied 61 SIDS and 34 control infants. They found the SIDS infants had significant changes in their brain stems and none were found in the controls. They stated:

> *Our findings indicate an immature development pattern of increased dendritic spine density in the SIDS brain stem, which may be responsible for abnormal central respiratory and arousal control. These significant quantitative differences in spine density are considered in the present study to represent an anatomical substrate of brainstem immaturity in the multifactorial pathogenesis of SIDS.*[71]

In other words they were saying this important anatomical finding links the brain stem to the cause of SIDS.

Pauli and others come so close to our ANVS theory that it is disappointing to think how many lives could have been saved if all infants born since they published this article (1984) had received an atlas examination by a chiropractor. We want to give you the entire abstract of "**Apnea and Sudden Unexpected Death in Infants with Achondroplasia,**" because of its importance. The critical area is in bold.

> *Thirteen infants with achondroplasia and sudden unexpected death or un-explained apnea were discovered through nonsystemic retrospective case collection. Most were initially thought to have died from sudden infant death syndrome. However, historical and pathologic findings suggest that many of these infants had **apnea and sudden unexpected death secondary to acute or chronic compression of the lower brainstem or cervical spinal cord.** Infants with achondroplasia evidently are at considerable increased risk for such deaths between 1 month and 1 year of age. Appropriate intervention, given these previously unrecognized risks, may include cervical restraint, polysomnographic evaluation, and apnea monitoring.[72]*

It is our opinion that the atlas vertebrae in these infants should be examined closely by a chiropractor and adjusted to remove the pressure on the brain stem and upper cervical spinal cord.

Another compelling paper that supports the Atlas VSC-SIDS Theory is, "**Cerebral Hypoperfusion in the Sudden Infant Death Syndrome? Brainstem Gliosis and Vasculature.**" We will quote the abstract written by Takashima and others:

> *Gliosis is increased in the respiratory control area of the brainstem in victims of sudden infant death syndrome (SIDS), as it is in infants who have died of congenital heart disease. In the latter, the lesions appear to result from hypoxia or ischemia, and studies of the brainstem microvasculature of SIDS victims indicated a close relationship between the gliosis and adjacent vasculature. It is postulated that cerebral hypoperfusion may play a role in SIDS.[73]*

The authors Bland and Emery in **"Unexpected Death of Children with Achondroplasia after the Perinatal Period"** suggested that death in children with achondroplasia appears to be related to brain stem lesions secondary to deformities of the foramen magnum and posterior fossa.[74] This supports the Atlas VSC Theory, in that we believe abnormal uterine constraint can cause deformities in the upper cervical area, including the foramen magnum (the opening in the base of the skull that the spinal cord passes through).

Nodar and others in their paper, "**Abnormal Brain Stem Potentials in Infants with Threatened Sudden Infant Death Syndrome**" studied 15 infants who were identified as being "at risk" for SIDS and tested them with BAEP techniques. All infants demonstrated abnormalities on two or more of the seven criteria employed to assess results. The data indicated that BAEP testing may play a significant role in the identification and monitoring of these children.[75]

Harrison in "**Infant Apnea Syndromes: Part II**" stated:

> *Subtle neurologic changes due to apnea, including those caused by hypoxia [decreased oxygen] and bradycardia [decreased heart rate] may be responsible for brain stem and cerebral dysfunction. These dysfunctions may be*

related to a higher risk for SIDS or long term minor neurologic problems. Further studies are recommended to evaluate the relationship between apnea-related infant morbidity and oxygenation of the brain.[76]

Thus, according to Dr. Harrison, there appears to be a link between lack of oxygen to the brain stem (which implicates the vertebral arteries, which can be compromised when an Atlas VSC is present) and **SIDS, or minor long term neurologic problems.** We want to stress this point, as we are not only interested in reducing SIDS, but improving the health of infants. Chiropractors have been saying for years that by removing subluxations, the function of the nerve system is improved. If the subluxation remains, a number of neurologic consequences can take place, either major or minor.

One of our favorite papers was written by Drs. Kinney and Filiano. "**Brainstem Research in Sudden Infant Death Syndrome**" was written for pediatricians, and provided an overview of SIDS brain stem research. The stated,

> *One of the leading hypotheses in SIDS research is that SIDS is due to a subtle defect in brainstem and neural circuits that control respiration and/ or cardiac stability during sleep. The rationale for the brainstem hypotheses and possible mechanisms of sleep-related sudden death is reviewed. The neuropathological studies of SIDS in the context of the neuroanatomy and neurochemistry of cardiorespiration and arousal are summarized. Quantitative abnormalities in brainstem reactive astrocytes (scar cells), dendritic spines, and neurotransmitter levels, and the number of small myelinated vagal fibers have been reported in SIDS. The cause of these abnormalities is unknown, and their relationship to each other or sudden death is unclear. Their complete elucidation, however, is perhaps the most compelling reason for **SIDS brainstem research, since such abnormalities could be the critical clues necessary for solving SIDS.**[77]*

The following information was an update recently placed on the Web site of Children's Hospital in Boston. It reinforces the SIDS-brain stem connection.

> *Hannah Kinney, a senior MRRC (Mental Retardation Research Center) investigator in the Basic Neuroscience Program, has discovered a specific defect in muscarinic receptors in the arcuate nucleus of infants dying with sudden infant death syndrome (SIDS). This observation is of extraordinary importance because the arcuate nucleus mediates the cardiorespiratory response to hypercarbia and asphyxia, insults considered important in the genesis of SIDS in various clinical settings, e.g., prone sleeping position. These observations may have finally defined the defect that makes certain infants vulnerable to SIDS at the critical periods of neurologic and neurophysiologic development early in the first year of life. Means of identification of the defect in muscarinic receptors in the living infant could lead to measures to prevent SIDS in such vulnerable infants. (www.tch.harvard.edu/neurology/hkres.html Children's Hospital, Boston. Mental Retardation Research Center, 300 Longwood Ave, Boston, MA 02115. March 1998)*

In "**Neglected Spinal Cord, Brain Stem and Musculoskeletal Injuries Stemming From Birth Trauma,**" Dr. Gottlieb reviewed the medical literature to determine the cause, diagnosis, prognosis, treatment, and prevention of injuries resulting from birth trauma. The review included case studies and other review articles on birth injuries to the spinal cord, brain stem, brachial plexus, skull, vertebrae, clavicle, and other parts of the neural and musculoskeletal systems. The abstract of the paper stated,

Birth injuries can have a wide range of deleterious effects, including respiratory depression or distress, vascular compromise, various palsies, paralysis, spinal deformities, failure to thrive, sleeping and eating disorders, lowered immune resistance, tonsillitis, enteritis, otitis, colic, and torticollis. Damage to the reticular nuclei just dorsal to the inferior olives of the brain stem can cause respiratory depression, which accounts for a large percentage of neonatal deaths, and damage to the vagus nerve may play a role in another type of infant death, Sudden Infant Death Syndrome (SIDS). The vagus nerve has been implicated in SIDS because it regulates tidal volume, respiratory rate, and respiratory reflexes. It is postulated that vagal damage modifies the permeability of the lung capillaries so the plasma leaves the pulmonary vessels on a scale so large that edema of the lungs results. Damage to the vagus nerve also can alter cardiac rhythm. Changes in obstetric techniques could prevent many stillbirths and birth injuries. However, even obstetric specialists cannot agree on which techniques are safest. Many birth traumas are not reparable, either surgically or non-surgically. But some conditions respond favorably to non-surgical treatment, including spinal cord joint fixations, blockages, and minor dislocations. Specialists in chiropractic are trained to find these impairments of mobility and treat them with adjustments or manipulations. In one case study of a 10-month old girl who suffered torticollis from birth after suction delivery, skull and facial asymmetry developed and the baby could not sit or crawl. The infant was found to have a moderate dislocation of the occiput, which was given manual impulse treatment. After two treatments, most of the infant's symptoms had disappeared and she exhibited normal development. Chiropractic manipulation is a valuable resource for treating musculoskeletal insults in the neonate and infant.[78]

The previous paper emphasizes what we as Chiropractic Atlas Orthogonists are saying; trauma during the birth process to the brain stem and the upper cervical spine can result in nerve and spinal cord damage. We believe all children should have their atlas checked by a qualified chiropractor. Birth trauma may be silent and not easy to recognize but the effects may be severe and irreversible if not detected and corrected through an atlas adjustment shortly after birth.

Doctors Korbkin and Guilleminault as part of the Sudden Infant Death Research Project at Stanford University School of Medicine, published a paper that supports a chiropractic-SIDS relationship. Although they did not directly implicate the brain stem, we would like to mention their study here. The researchers performed neurological examinations on forty-one infants that had a "near miss incident," seven normal siblings of babies who died of SIDS and twenty-one normal control infants. They found that near-miss infants under three months of age had consistent abnormalities of muscle tone, particularly shoulder hypotonia (abnormal muscle tone). These abnormalities disappeared with maturation, but only sixty percent of older infants who had suffered near miss episodes were neurologically and developmentally normal. The authors stated, "Thus, infants who present with near miss episodes may have an underlying central nervous system abnormality or may acquire some abnormality as a result of the episode." [79]

We believe this abnormality can be traced to the atlas vertebral subluxation complex! If you ask, "How can some of these abnormalities disappear with age (or maturation as the paper stated)?" The answer is, "We know the body is an amazing healing being and it is going to do whatever it can to heal and overcome any obstacle and abnormality." What is very interesting however, is that the researchers found that **forty percent of the children that were followed had measurable neurological and developmental problems**. So the body can overcome many challenges, but these doctors found that 40% of the time long-term neurological problems may remain.

The final paper we will mention in this section is titled "**Red Nucleus inhibits Breathing during Hypoxia in Neonates**," written by Drs. Ackland, Noble and Hanson.[80] The red nucleus is an area in the brain stem and part of the reticular formation which controls several functions. In their paper, the authors note that the response to acute hypoxia is an initial increase in breathing followed by a fall to or below normal. They present evidence from brain stem and peripheral chemoreflex studies supporting the concept that in addition to the peripheral chemoreceptors, hypoxia also activates brain stem pathways that **inhibit ventilation**. A key part of the inhibitory pathway is an area within the red nucleus. The researchers found that when they destroyed the red nucleus in rabbits, there was no longer a decrease in ventilation during low blood oxygen levels (which typically takes place) stated:

> *Destruction of this area in young decerebrate rabbits abolishes the ventilatory fall during hypoxia, yet has no effect on respiratory control during normoxia and does not affect arterial blood pressure changes in hypoxia. In support of this hypothesis, we report that there are neurones within the red nucleus that increase their discharge in hypoxia.*

They discuss the role of higher brain stem/hypothalamic (higher brain tissue) function in central respiratory control during hypoxia in the fetus and neonate. The point we want to stress by mentioning this paper is that low oxygen levels at the brain stem (hypothetically caused by Atlas VSC) can inhibit respiration.

The previous papers offer compelling evidence that a brain stem-SIDS correlation exists. As we stated earlier, there are well over 100 scientific research papers that point to the brain stem as a critical link to SIDS. Researchers have done an excellent job setting the stage for the Atlas VSC-SIDS Theory.

In Section I of this chapter we introduced three theories that may explain how an Atlas subluxation complex can affect the brain stem. Again they are:

1. The Dentate Ligament Cord Distortion Hypothesis (DLCDH)

2. The Proprioceptive Insult Hypothesis

3. The Vertebral Artery Ischemia Theory

The following pages contain more detail about these three theories. Again, this area is primarily written for the individual with a knowledge of anatomy and physiology.

1. THE DENTATE LIGAMENT CORD DISTORTION HYPOTHESIS (DLCDH)

The DLCDH utilizes the unique anatomy of the upper cervical spine to provide a model that explains how a misalignment of the atlas can produce neurological insult directly via mechanical irritation of the spinal cord and brain stem, and indirectly via vascular compromise of the cervical cord. This hypothesis states that misalignments of the upper cervical vertebrae, because of their unique attachment to the spinal cord by means of the dentate ligaments, can directly stress and deform the spinal cord. Subsequently, this stress on the cord, in addition to direct mechanical irritation, may produce venous occlusion with stasis of blood and result in anoxia in particular areas of the upper cervical cord.[43]

Dr. Grostic, in his paper, "The Dentate Ligament Cord Distortion Hypothesis" stated:

> In addition to direct mechanical irritation of the tracts of the spinal cord, this mechanism may involve a vascular component. Gillilan, in an investigation of the venous drainage system of the cervical spinal cord, observed that the small radicular veins of the upper cervical cord were not as redundant as those elsewhere in the spinal cord and that mechanical obstruction of the veins could cause stasis of blood and ischemia in the portion of the spinal cord drained by these veins. She noted that venous stasis would tend to cause ischemia first in the lateral columns of the cord. Gillilan pointed out that because these veins operate at such low pressures, they are easily occluded by compressive forces. She further noted that the dentate ligament may be one means of transmitting mechanical stresses to the cord.

> Important to this proposed model is that ischemia first increases the irritability of nerves. Thus, a purely mechanical irritation of the nerve tracts may be aggravated by localized ischemia and increased sensitivity to the effects of mechanical irritation.

As we stated earlier, it is our opinion that this may be one cause of the malformations, immaturity and gliosis that are frequently found in the brain stem of SIDS victims upon autopsy as reported by many authors including Dr. Hannah Kinney.[81] It may also be the reason for demyelination found in vagus nerves of many SIDS victims. The vagus nerve has also been implicated in SIDS because it regulates tidal volume, respiratory rate and reflexes, and alters cardiac rhythm.[78]

2. THE PROPRIOCEPTIVE INSULT HYPOTHESIS

Doctors Kleinman and Crowe stated, "Factual evidence strongly suggests that the atlas adjustment has an effect on the entire nervous system primarily through its effect on joint mechanoreceptors." They went on to say, "The most important proprioceptive information needed for maintenance of equilibrium is derived from the joint receptors of the upper cervical spine, appraising the orientation of the head in respect to the body."[46] They suggested that an upper cervical misalignment can adversely affect reticular formation activity by abnormal afferentation to the thalamus.

> The reticular formation is a vital center of regulatory nuclei, termed a formation because its cell bodies are widespread within the tegmentum of the medulla, pons and midbrain. The neurons of the reticular formation provide a

large network of synaptic activity directed both rostrally and caudally along the brainstem.

The reticular formation is responsible for body homeostasis including:

1. The direct regulation of posture by inhibition and facilitation of synergistic and antagonistic muscle groups, ipsilaterally and contralaterally.

2. ***Direct regulation of autonomic response.***

3. Direct regulation of consciousness, wakefulness and pain as well.[46]

Dr. Speransky stated,

> *The nervous system is an organ which cannot be altered locally. Local interference affects the whole nervous network: these changes pass away gradually and not completely, and give rise to a number of adaptations to the new artificial norm. The nervous system is now a new object, after the local lesion, and reacts to stimuli in a new fashion.*[82]

The previous quote helps explain the problem brought up by Dr. Kinney et al.[4] They stated that brains of SIDS victims can look "normal", as can those of profound mental retardation, seizure disorders, and schizophrenia patients, or at the most, contain trivial and nonspecific lesions by conventional histopathologic criteria.

The Autonomic Nervous System

This is the area of true importance for our research in finding answers to SIDS. The area of least research and yet great promise for health benefits derived from chiropractic care is the Autonomic Nervous System. This system controls the function of all organs including the heart, lungs, most glands and smooth muscle. The sympathetic (SNS) and parasympathetic (PNS) nervous systems, with two or three exceptions, supply the same organs or tissues but are antagonistic in nature. For instance, the SNS will dilate the pupils and the PNS will constrict them.

A Connection between the Autonomic Nervous System and the Cervical Spine

Neuroscience is proving that structural integrity, particularly that of the upper cervical spine, with its various intimate relationships with several neural components has a direct influence on the nervous system's assessment and coordination of whole body function, mainly health.

One area that we find very interesting is the connection of the **locus ceruleus** to the cervical spine. The locus ceruleus is located near the periventricular gray of the upper part of the fourth ventricle and is an irregular collection of pigmented cells. It is a very tiny nuclei of the reticular system. It is very interesting that it has a direct connection to the cervical spine because there are connections from the locus ceruleus to the telencephalon, the diencephalon, the brain stem, the midbrain, the pons and the medulla, the cerebellum as well as the spinal cord.[83]

Although the locus ceruleus is a relatively small structure, it can be identified readily in gross sections of the brain stem. Cells of this nucleus are partially intermingled with those of the mesencephalic nucleus of the trigeminal nerve, but the large globular neurons of the mesencephalic nucleus extend further dorsally and rostrally at the margin of the central gray. Cells of the locus ceruleus are of two types:

1. Medium-sized cells with eccentric nuclei containing clumps of melanin pigment granules and

2. Small oval cells with scant cytoplasm and no pigment. Ventrolateral to the locus ceruleus is a diffuse collection of similar cells known as the nucleus subceruleus.[86]

The significance of this small pigmented nucleus (the locus ceruleus) remained unknown until it was demonstrated by a sensitive flourescence technique that its cells contain catecholamines, nearly all of which are norepinephrine. Unlike other brain stem norepinephrine cells found as scattered neurons in the lateral tegmentum, the locus ceruleus is a compact nucleus that projects fibers to the telencephalon, diencephalon, midbrain, cerebellum, pons, medulla, and spinal cord.[84] The interesting thing is that the locus ceruleus, with its norepinephrine, is sending information directly to the thalamus without synaptic activity. It is almost like the adrenal medulla that gets direct adrenaline from the autonomic nervous system.

To summarize about the tiny locus ceruleus, it literally affects every part of the brain, and also has direct effects on the lateral hypothalamus, which drives the Autonomic Nervous System. It is also now thought to have direct activity on different organ systems in the body. *Because the locus ceruleus and subceruleus project fibers down to spinal levels we believe this may be a key to the chiropractic link to influencing brain function.*

Here is another interesting fact for the Atlas VSC-SIDS Theory (from *Carpenter's Neuroanatomy*), "The locus ceruleus and its efferent projections have been considered to **play a role in paradoxical sleep, facilitation and inhibition of sensory neurons, and control of cortical activation.**"[84] Paradoxical sleep has several characteristics, a few of which include a reduction in blood pressure, bradycardia and irregular respirations. "In addition, descending noradrenergic fibers from the locus ceruleus may supply preganglionic sympathetic neurons in the intermediolateral cell column at the thoracic and upper lumbar levels." (This means there are further effects on the cardiovascular system.)

3. THE VERTEBRAL ARTERY ISCHEMIA THEORY

The Vertebral Artery Ischemia Theory is the third explanation of how an atlas subluxation complex can affect the brain stem. The vertebral arteries, which ascend through the foramina transversaria of C6 through C1 bilaterally, supply blood to the brain stem and other critical brain centers. When the cervical spine is excessively axially rotated, symptoms of nausea, vertigo, tinnitus, and visual disturbances can be present due to occlusion of the vertebral artery.[86] Since the vagus nerve has its nuclei in the brain stem, if there is vertebral artery ischemia, the vagus nerve can be adversely affected, thus disturbing normal respiration and cardiac function. Dr. Roy Sweat, the founder of the Atlas Orthogonal Procedure, stated when there is rotation between the atlas and axis of 15 degrees or more, this can cause vertebral artery ischemia.[86] With many births, the physician or attendant will rotate the infant's head to help the delivery process. This head rotation may be the first cause of Atlas VSC and Atlas Neuro-Vascular Syndrome, and the first step in the malfunctioning of the brain stem and vagus nerve.

Doctors Roy Sweat and Thomas Sievert wrote a paper titled **"Chiropractic and the Vertebral Arteries"** that details this relationship.[47] Because their paper explains the importance of the vertebral arteries so well, we quote it liberally so that the relevance between the vertebral arteries and SIDS can be understood.

> *The fundamentals of the chiropractic profession are based on vertebral and osseous involvement's producing neurological insult and disease. Now we have a circulatory fundamental with vertebral and osseous involvement producing vertebral artery insult resulting in ischemia, causing neurological deficit and disease. A variety of diseases, maladies and symptomatic conditions in which the chiropractic profession has achieved outstanding success and miraculous results, can now be documented by the medical profession as related to vertebral artery insult.*

> *Central peripheral nervous system dysfunctions due to vertebral artery compromise have been described by researchers to occur from degenerative, traumatic, and kinematic effects, and from subluxations of the cervical spine. These findings broaden the spectrum of chiropractic treatment to provide for the removal of vascular compromise as well as neurological insult. This current evidence is an important explanation of the effectiveness of chiropractic care for the treatment of cranial nerve, brain stem, cerebellum, and posterior cerebral functional disorders.*

> *The vertebral artery is the major source of blood supply to the cervical spinal cord and brain stem which includes the medulla oblongata, pons, and midbrain. It also supplies the visual cortex of the cerebrum and the cerebellum via the basilar artery. Compression of the vertebral artery has been noted by numerous authorities and is reported to produce a variety of bizarre symptoms resulting from ischemia. Minor compromise of the arterial blood flow is characterized by Barr-Lieou syndrome. Severe kinking of the vertebral artery may result in the formation of thrombosis that may extend superiorly and occlude the posterior inferior cerebellar artery producing Wallenberg's syndrome.*

> ### *Review of Literature*

> *Hadley states, "The vertebral artery is an important link in the collateral cerebral blood supply. The symptoms constitute a most bizarre and confusing clinical picture, which has been described as the Barr-Lieou syndrome. They include: headache, vertigo, nausea, vomiting, nystagmus and suboccipital tenderness."*

> *In their book titled,* The Cervical Spine, *published by the Cervical Spine Research Society of the medical profession, Ian MacNab states, "Minor degrees of vertebral artery compromise may be responsible for the so-called vertebral artery syndrome consisting of dizziness, tinnitus, intermittent blurring of vision*

and occasional episodes of retro-occular pain. Occasionally, a neurocentral osteophyte may produce severe kinking of the artery, resulting eventually in a vertebral artery thrombosis that may extend superiorly and involve the posteroinferior cerebellar artery. Occlusion of this artery leads to the development of Wallenberg's syndrome, which is associated with the following symptom complex.

1. *Dysphagia, ipsilateral palatal weakness, and vocal cord paralysis from involvement of the nucleus ambiguous of the vagus.*

2. *Impairment of sensation to pain and temperature on the same side of the face from involvement of the descending root and nucleus of the fifth nerve.*

3. *Horner's syndrome in the homolateral eye from the involvement of the descending sympathetic fibers.*

4. *Nystagmus due to the involvement of the vestibular nuclei.*

5. *Cerebellar dysfunction in the ipsilateral arm and leg from interference of the function of the midbrain and cerebellum.*

6. *Impairment of sensation to pain and temperature on the side of the body opposite from the involvement of the spinothalamic tract.*

Epstein states, "Spondylotic deformities may impinge on the foramina transversaria and cause compression of the vertebral artery, thereby producing a clinical syndrome of vascular insufficiency with headache, vertigo, visual and speech defects and gait impairment.

Von Torklus states, "Vascular disturbances (irritation of the vertebral arteries and the posterior cervical sympathetic plexus, commonly referred to as vertebralis syndrome can cause occlusion of the venous or cerebrospinal fluid circulation.

Kabat states, "Decreased blood flow in the basilar artery and the resulting ischemia of the brainstem, cerebellum and visual cortex produces a form of basilar artery syndrome. More common complaints from compression of the vertebral artery are vertigo, syncope, and nausea. Infrequent symptoms from such compression of the vertebral artery include impairment of vision, diminished sensation in the face, intention tremor or ataxia, and dysphagia. These different complaints usually occur singly but may appear together. Vertigo from compression of the vertebral artery is the result of ischemia of the brain stem affecting vestibular function. Diminished sensation in the face, usually unilateral and localized to the lips or around the orbit, is another manifestation of compression of the vertebral artery produced by ischemia of the sensory nucleus of the fifth cranial nerve in the pons. Light-headedness or feeling faint may be caused by compression of the vertebral artery. Compression of the vertebral artery produces ischemia of the brain stem, which can also affect the function of the vomiting center.

Rothman and Simeone state, "Children with occipitocervical anomalies may be more susceptible to vertebral artery injury and brain stem ischemia, particularly those who undergo skull traction for correction of scoliosis. Even moderate amounts of traction (less than 15 pounds) that normally would be well tolerated may compromise these abnormal vessels. Although this condi-

tion is congenital, many patients do not develop symptoms until the second or third decade of life".

Rothman and Simeone also state, "The vertebral arteries may be compressed in chronic cervical disc disease by three mechanisms that are obvious when one considers the anatomic confines of the foramen transversarium in vertebrae C2 through C6 through which the vertebral artery passes. These are (1) osteophytes from the lateral portion of the disc margin, (2) osteophytes extending anteriorly from the zygapophyseal joint and (3) compression by the inferior articular facet from posterior subluxation with scissoring action by the adjacent superior articulating facet."

White and Panjabi state, "There is extensive axial rotation between C1 and C2. Studies have shown that 50 percent of axial rotation in the neck occurs at C1-C2 and that the remainder occurs at the joints of the lower cervical spine. The extensive amount (47 degrees) of axial (y-axis) rotation at C1-C2 can sometimes cause clinical problems with the vertebral artery. Symptoms of vertigo, nausea, tinnitus and visual disturbances may occur from occlusion of the vertebral artery associated with axial rotation of the atlas".

At the conclusion of part one of their paper, Doctors Sweat and Sievert stated, "Chiropractic care of the cervical spine for vertibrobasilar symptomatology is necessary and extremely successful."

In part two of their paper, the doctors describe the mechanisms for compression in the vertebral arteries. The main reason for vulnerability of the vertebral arteries to compressive forces is that it is so tortuous in the upper cervical spine. More specifically, due to the fact that the vertebral artery makes four right angle turns in the area of 20 to 30 millimeters, from the transverse process of the second cervical vertebra to the occiput. They went on to state:

> *. . . the mechanisms of compression of the vertebral artery can occur by extremes of rotation and extension, hyperplastic posterior joints, neurocentral osteophytes, herniation of the nucleus pulposus and* **subluxations.**

> *Salecki studied the effect of the large rotational movements of C1-C2 on the vertebral artery and found that 30 degrees of rotation produced kinking accompanied by stretching of the contralateral artery, which becomes more marked as the angle of rotation is increased. He also found that at 45 degrees rotation the ipsilateral vertebral artery begins to kink. If blood flow is significantly decreased, symptoms of ischemia may be elicited.[47]*

In addition to the methods of vertebral artery compromise that doctors Sweat and Sievert mention, we believe there is another important connection between atlas subluxations and vertebral artery compromise. Dr. Seletz stated in the *Journal of the American Medical Association* in 1958,

> *The vertebral nerve lies within the transverse foramina and travels alongside the vertebral artery. The vertebral nerve originates from the stellate ganglion and supplies the vertebral and basilar vessels. Injury to this nerve produces spasm of the vertebral arteries and gives rise to disturbed circulation to the pons and portions of the medulla containing the nuclei or origin of the lower seven cranial nerves. . . .[87]*

In other words, damage (or interference) to the nerves in this area (Atlas VSC) may cause vertebral artery ischemia, resulting in brain stem dysfunction.

Research Papers Implicating the Vertebral Arteries in SIDS

A group of researchers from Australia recently published a paper that suggests vertebral artery compression during sleep may be a contributing factor in sudden infant death syndrome. They stated:

> *Vertebral artery compression causing brainstem ischemia has been suggested to underlie the sudden infant death syndrome. Vertebral artery distortion from neck movements has been demonstrated by angiography in infants, but direct evidence for arterial compression is lacking.*[88]

The researchers studied the arteries of twenty infants that died of SIDS and other causes. They examined five cases with the neck in the extended position, nine cases where the head was rotated ninety degrees to the right, and six cases where the neck was held in the neutral position. What they found was that in **three of the five extended cases**, bilateral vertebral artery compression was seen between the occipital bone and the atlas (C1). In three of nine rotated cases, the left vertebral artery was compressed adjacent to C1 before the artery entered the transverse foramen. No vertebral artery compression was seen in the necks held in the neutral position.

They concluded by stating:

> *The vertebral arteries of some infants can be compressed by neck movement. This could induce lethal brainstem ischemia in infants with inadequate collateral blood flow or with poor compensatory arterial dilatation, and may underlie some cases of sudden infant death syndrome.*[88]

We believe and hope to demonstrate through research projects that by keeping an infant's atlas in proper alignment, compression of the vertebral arteries and abnormal blood supply to the brain stem can be avoided. If this can be demonstrated, it stands to reason that through atlas correction, normal function of the brain stem may be maintained.

In an earlier paper written by two of the same researchers from Australia titled, "**Vulnerability of the infant brain stem to ischemia: a possible cause of sudden infant death syndrome,**" Drs. Pamphlett and Murray examined arteries that supply blood to the brain and how extension and rotation of the head affected blood flow through these arteries. What they found was that there was a significant difference in conduction of blood flow in vertebral arteries from one side to the other and that head movement can decrease the blood supply to the brain stem:

> *In conclusion, the lag in available blood flow and small communicating and asymmetric vertebral arteries may predispose the infant brain stem to ischemia if one or both vertebral arteries are occluded by head rotation or extension. Because these head movements are likely to be accentuated in the prone sleeping position (a risk factor for sudden infant death syndrome), we suggest that vertebral artery occlusion may underlie some cases of sudden unexpected infant death.*[89]

Doctors Saternus and Adam also found head rotation to decrease vertebral artery blood flow.[90]

Additional research papers have been published that link compromise of the vertebral arteries and brain stem malfunction.[91-94] Most of these papers have to do with head position. Some used doppler ultrasound to document the findings. One of the papers noted:

> *The reduction of the blood flow is caused by compression of the contralateral vertebral artery at the craniocervical junction. CONCLUSION: The reduction of blood flow in the VA [vertebral arteries] and especially the BA [basilar artery] may cause hypoperfusion of the brainstem followed by central brady-cardia and apnea. Hypoperfusion of the brainstem in dependence on head and body position may be a significant cause of SIDS.*[94]

The craniocervical junction is the atlas area. Therefore, we suggest this critical area be examined closely to make sure no stress, strain, tight musculature, or irritated nerves are present, which could adversely affect the vertebral arteries, as the brain stem is dependent on the blood supplied by them.

We hypothesize that, as these researchers have suggested, vertebral artery occlusion through rotation of the head can cause SIDS; therefore rotation of the atlas (Atlas VSC) may cause abnormal blood flow through the vertebral arteries and in some infants this may result in SIDS.

We have presented three theories that explain how an atlas subluxation can cause brain stem neurological insult. We believe these theories may work independently, or in conjunction with each other to cause brain stem dysfunction. As many researchers have found the brain stem to play a critical role in SIDS, it would be prudent to have an infant's atlas examined by a chiropractor. We believe more research needs to be performed that shows the effects of atlas correction on brain stem function and different areas of infant health.

Chiropractic Success with Possible "SIDS-Related" Symptoms

Although some researchers consider apnea (when infants stop breathing) to not be a leading indicator of SIDS, we feel the research performed by Dr. Ronald Harper and his team at the University of California at Los Angeles (UCLA), who found abnormal respiratory control in infants who later died of SIDS, to be extremely important.[1] We present these case studies to support our theory that chiropractic can have dramatic effects on respiratory function.

Case Study #1

KB, a female born 8 pounds on February 9, 1990 to a healthy, twenty two-year-old married caucasian mother. KB was the first born, and was a cephalic presentation of a vaginal delivery. Labor and delivery were unremarkable, however "low forceps" were used. She had spontaneous respiration and oxygen was given. At both one and five minutes, she had an Apgar score of 9. No medication was administered and no observed abnormalities were present.

At three days old KB had an apnea episode (stopped breathing), and became cyanotic (turned blue) while being held by the mother. The mother called 911. KB was resuscitated and taken to a hospital. There she was examined by a pediatric neurologist and fitted for a respiratory monitor. Within a period of 48 hours she had 111 apnea attacks. Diagnosis was sleep apnea due to reflux and surgery was suggested for the gastric sphincter. The parents decided against the surgery. KB was released and parents were instructed to use the apnea monitor for one year and have periodic re-evaluations with the neurologist.

On February 26, 1990 at two and one half weeks old, KB was presented for chiropractic care at the Sweat Chiropractic Clinic for Atlas Orthogonality. The mother stated KB had 7 apnea attacks the previous day. A complete history and chiropractic examination including leg check and scanning palpation according to Atlas Orthogonal Chiropractic Procedures were performed.[2] Clinical signs of an upper cervical subluxation were present. Cervical x-rays following the Atlas Orthogonal Chiropractic Procedure were taken to determine line of correction necessary to adjust the subluxation.[3] X-ray analysis was performed according to Atlas Orthogonal Chiropractic Procedures.[4] The patient was then adjusted with the Atlas Orthogonal Percussion Instrument and post x-rays were taken to determine extent of correction.[5, 3]

The following day, February 27, KB was again examined and was found to be in adjustment using the Atlas Orthogonal Chiropractic criteria. KB's mother reported one apnea attack the previous night.

On March 1, 1990 KB was examined. She had had two apnea attacks the previous night. Examination revealed patient to be out of adjustment. Patient was re-adjusted with the Atlas Orthogonal Percussion Instrument.

From March 9, 1990 to April 5, 1990 she maintained her adjustment and had only two apnea attacks.

May 2, 1990 she was examined again and did not need an adjustment and mother reported one attack since previous visit.

On June 5, 1990 the neurologist examined KB and the monitor was removed (eight months before the previously suggested time frame of one year).

April 16, 1991 KB returned for a chiropractic check up. She had maintained her adjustment for over one year and no neurologic involvement was present.

Case Study #2

AG, a male born 7 pounds on June 1, 1996 to a healthy, thirty-two-year-old married Caucasian mother. AG was the first born, and was a cephalic presentation of a vaginal delivery. The mother was induced because she was told she was "overdue" by one week. Induction consisted of a cervical prostaglandin gel suppository. Because labor did not begin after the first application of the gel, it was given a second time, four hours later. The labor lasted twenty-four hours from the beginning of the administration of the gel until delivery. Upon delivery, AG was delayed in breathing and oxygen was given.

At two days old, when arriving home from the hospital, AG stopped breathing and turned blue. Upon picking him up, AG began breathing again. The parents reported that AG seemed to have a difficult time breathing over the next few days.

At five days old his mother brought AG to the office of Specific Chiropractic for an evaluation and treatment. A complete history and chiropractic examination including leg check and scanning palpation according to Atlas Orthogonal Chiropractic Procedures was performed.[2, 5] Clinical signs of an upper cervical subluxation were present. Cervical x-rays following the Atlas Orthogonal Chiropractic Procedure

71

were taken to determine line of correction necessary to adjust the subluxation.[3] X-ray analysis was performed according to the Atlas Orthogonal Chiropractic Procedure (4). The patient was then adjusted with the Atlas Orthogonal Percussion Instrument and post x-rays were taken to determine extent of correction. After the first adjustment, AG did not have another apnea episode.

AG has been checked and adjusted as needed for atlas subluxations for the past four years. Chiropractic has been a regular part of his healthcare and has helped him maintain excellent health with little medication and low incidence of illness.

Although these are just two case studies, and they are not compared to a control group, we believe they are good examples of apnea responding to Atlas VSC correction. We hope these cases raise the public's awareness that an infant's atlas needs to be examined, and adjusted if necessary, to ensure optimum health.

6

Avoiding Shaken Baby Syndrome and Other Infant Trauma

Shaken baby syndrome is a tragic injury to an infant that usually takes place after an adult has lost his or her temper with that infant, and shakes the baby to try to make it stop crying. Frequently, the reason for the loss of control from the parent or caregiver, is due to inconsolable crying by the infant, also called colic. In this chapter, we explain how a healthy baby is a happy baby, and how chiropractic care can reduce colic, and therefore the incidence of shaken baby syndrome.

The following information was taken from a media advisory published by the SIDS Alliance titled "Differentiating Between Sudden Infant Death Syndrome, Shaken Baby Syndrome, and Accidental Infant Deaths Associated with Bedsharing."

*Shaken Baby Syndrome (SBS) is an acquired traumatic brain injury caused when a frustrated adult "shakes" a child, usually less than one year of age but as old as five, in order to stop them from crying. Other triggering events include toilet training difficulties and feeding problems. While there are no scientific studies in existence which document the amount of force causing serious injury through shaking of an infant, it is evident that babies' neck muscles are too weak to support their disproportionately large, heavy heads. When shaking occurs, the brain bounces within the skull cavity, bruising the brain tissue. The brain then swells, creating pressure and leading to bleeding within the skull. As a result, the infant may experience seizures, limpness of the arms or legs, excessive drooling, and the heart or breathing may stop resulting in death. SBS is considered a serious form of child abuse. **With an autopsy, it is virtually impossible to mask SBS as SIDS.**

Physicians often report possible SBS when a child is brought in for medical attention due to falls, difficulty breathing, seizures, vomiting, altered consciousness or choking. The caregiver may report that the baby was shaken in an effort* *to resuscitate it. To diagnose SBS, physicians look for retinal bleeding, blood in the brain, and increased head size indicating excessive accumulation of fluid in the brain. Damage to the spinal cord and broken ribs from grasping the baby too hard are other signals of SBS. According to child abuse experts there are about 1,000 cases in the U.S. in which SBS claims an infant's life each year; **cases in which infants are injured are more common.** Adult males in their early 20's who are the baby's father or the mother's boyfriend constitute 65-90% of the perpetrators. Females who injure babies by shaking them are more likely to be baby-sitters or child-care providers than mothers.*[1]

From the disturbing previous two paragraphs, it must be stressed to parents and any adult who is going to be in contact with infants the need to be aware of some basic spinal hygiene rules. Many adults lack the awareness of the critical anatomy and the possible damage that can be done to an infant's spine if handled improperly. Parents need to treat the infant's head and neck more delicately than a china doll. Very few new parents are actually taught how to properly handle a baby. It must be stressed to parents that if they ever feel frustrated and angry for whatever reason to never take it out by shaking an infant. The results can be devastating and often irreversible.

A two or three-year-old sibling of an infant does not understand the baby is not a doll and cannot be tugged, pulled, shaken or dragged across the floor. Adults need to emphasize to the new big brother or sister the importance of being gentle, and must put these words into practice to ensure that careless handling does not damage a newborn's vital nervous system.

Sometimes even doctors, midwives and nurses need to be reminded

Understandably, the goal of an obstetrical team is to deliver a healthy baby, however some maneuvers often result in damaging or compromising an infant's spine and nerve system. We have spoken to many obstetrical nurses and have personally witnessed the lack of care and even force given to the infant's spine. They are handled almost in a violent fashion, the way they are flopped over from their backs to their stomachs so that the team can clean the newborn and perform the other procedures. Through educating the public on how important it is to handle a baby's spine with the utmost care, we hope that parents will have their newborn's neck examined for damaging subluxations as a regular part of their healthcare program.

Whiplash—Atlas Trauma

To stress the significance of potential injuries from shaking a baby, we want to explain what happens to the spine when whiplash takes place. In 1989 Dr. S.S. Neel wrote an article titled "Whiplash—Atlanto-Axial Trauma" that explains this injury in adults. It should not be difficult to understand that since an infant's head is disproportionately larger than that of an adult, its spine is much more susceptible to injury. Although the article may be difficult for some to understand due to the anatomy discussed, we would like to include it here:

Trauma to the atlanto-axial region following whiplash is a frequent yet "silent" finding. Due to straightening of the lordotic cervical curvature and the resultant degenerative changes of the C5–C6 disc spaces, emphasis is frequently placed on these radiographic findings and region. In other cases in clinical practice, it is frequently seen that patients will continue to present with bizarre symptoms with no "objective" findings. These patients continue to have upper back/neck spasms, headaches, nausea, and other complaints without reportable "objective" signs. These patients are victims of "upper cervical trauma."

Dr. B.J. Palmer was quick to state that the "upper cervical" region is the key to all disease. The upper cervical region may be the hidden key to common yet prolonged symptomatic changes following whiplash.

Wry neck and pain is a common complaint following whiplash. On examination, the muscles in the suboccipital area, the trapezius and sternocleidomastoid (S.C.M.) are involved. This frequently results from irritation of filaments of the spinal accessory nerve along the origin from the upper cervical portion of the spinal cord. The spinal accessory nerve supplies innervation to the S.C.M. and trapezius muscles.

Rotational hyperextension/hyperflexion injuries often cause compression of the vertebral arteries in the C1-2 region. This in turn influences other regions directly and indirectly, resulting in symptomatic changes. The most frequent confusing symptoms following such trauma may include vertigo (dizziness), diplopia (double vision), dysphagia (difficulty swallowing), ataxia (imbalance), disturbance in speech, syncope (fainting spells), nystagmus (involuntary lateral movement of the eyes), and Horner's syndrome." These are frequent symptoms associated with vertebral artery problems.

The C2 nerve is prone to injury since in its peculiar anatomy it is not protected posteriorly by pedicles or facets as are all the other nerve roots in the vertebral spine. Stretching injury to this region often gives rise to migraine-like headaches of hemicranial and orbital pain. Neurological dysfunction of the hypoglosial and trigeminal nerves is a common finding in such cases. Tentorial nerves originate from the first division of the trigeminal, while the dura on the anterior surface of the posterior fossa is supplied by the sensory portion of C2. Immediately following injury the patient complains of sensitivity changes in the jaw, ear, posterior portions of the upper neck and occiput.

Stretching of the vagal nerve fibers as it exits the cranium, in close proximity to the C1 vertebra, will create a noxious reflex which may create a chronic state of nausea.

*Clinically, it has been observed that direct or indirect whiplash injuries to the atlanto-axial junction influence the integrity and function of the neurovascular systems. **Prompt attention must be directed to the C1-2 [atlas] region to restore the functional dynamics of this region.**[2]*

Whiplash can occur in an infant if it is shaken, tossed, bounced, or if it falls onto its back, bottom, stomach, neck or head. We want to reiterate that although it may seem obvious to most people, infants must be handled with extreme care and every precaution should be taken to protect the infant from falls and other potential traumas. Childhood consists of many unavoidable falls, accidents and traumas. To most parents many of these injuries are brushed aside especially if there are no broken bones or bleeding. However the spine is often misaligned which may lead to damaging long-term health effects which are often over looked. As the great inventor Thomas Edison once said, "The doctor of the future will give no medicine, but interest his patients in the care of the human frame."

Preventing Colic (and its connection to Shaken Baby Syndrome)

The main reason we included the topic of Shaken Baby Syndrome in this book is because we want to raise awareness that if more infants were under chiropractic care there might be fewer cases of Shaken Baby Syndrome. This conclusion can be drawn by the fact that most cases of SBS are a result of a frustrated adult who loses his or her temper due to the inconsolable crying of the infant. This crying is often diagnosed as "colic." There have been several research studies performed and published that show that chiropractic care is effective for infants with colic. In one study, **a satisfactory result occurred within two weeks in 94% of the cases receiving chiropractic care**. Fifty-one percent of these infants had prior, unsuccessful treatment, usually drug therapy.[3] *Ninety-four percent,* that is an amazing result!

In another case study, a 3-month-old female suffered from colic with sleep interruption and appetite decrease. Chiropractic spinal adjustments on the infant helped improve the symptoms greatly. The results were obtained from direct observation and involvement of both parents and from interviews at each treatment. Specific adjustments to T7 and the upper cervical area relieved symptoms of infantile colic in a relatively short period of time. The patient received three adjustments with approximately a two-week period of time in between adjustments.[4]

An additional investigation into the effectiveness of chiropractic on colic involved a survey of the parents of 132 infants with colic. Following chiropractic adjustments, 91% of the parents reported an improvement, which occurred after an average of two to three adjustments, or one week after the treatment had begun.[5]

The first retrospective chiropractic study on treating colic was conducted in 1985, followed by a prospective multi-center study in 1989. Both of these studies suggest that chiropractic treatment had a positive effect on infantile colic, but since neither study had a control group, it was impossible to assess whether the chiropractic treatments were significantly better than placebo.

A study in the October 1999 *Journal of Manipulative and Physiological Therapeutics* has clearly demonstrated that chiropractic adjustments are superior to any other form of care for infantile colic.[6] The Danish National Health Service recruited 50 infants meeting the criteria for colic. After they were reviewed and monitored, they were randomly assigned to two groups:

1. Dimethicone (drug treatment) daily for two weeks

2. Spinal manipulation for two weeks by a local chiropractor.

The 25 infants under chiropractic care received an average of 3.8 adjustments. During the two-week treatments, the parents kept a colic diary in which they measured the daily hours of crying, and nurses visited the families to administer a weekly "infantile colic behavior profile." The results were:

- On days 4–7, hours of crying were reduced by 1 hour in the dimethicone group compared to a reduction of 2.4 hours in the chiropractic group (p=.04).

- On days 8–11, crying was reduced by 1 hour for the dimethicone group whereas the chiropractic group was reduced by 2.7 hours (p=.004).

The dimethicone group would have fared much worse than these results suggest if not for the dropout rate of the medicated group. All 25 infants in the manipulation group completed the 13 days of treatment, but there were nine dropouts in the dimethicone group: five dropped out before the first week's diary could be completed, and thus there was no data on the hours of crying for those five subjects. But the study did register the subjective evaluation of four of the five in the dimethicone group that quit in the first week: two described their child's condition as "worsened" and two others described it as "much worsened." Had these four infants completed the study, they would have significantly affected the limited positive effect of dimethicone. To quote the authors: "By excluding data from the dropouts, we are excluding more severe cases from the dimethicone group, and this has the effect of making that group appear better than it actually was." The authors make another comment that speaks directly to the issue:

Spinal manipulation is normally used in the treatment of musculoskeletal disorders, and the results of this trial leave open two possible interpretations. Either spinal manipulation is effective in the treatment of the visceral disorder infantile colic or infantile colic is, in fact, a musculoskeletal disorder, and not, as normally assumed, visceral. This study does not address this issue.

In summary, chiropractic reduced infants' crying from an average of 3.9 hours per day to just over one hour per day. That is nearly a 75% improvement. This is exciting news for parents who have infants with colic and for the pediatricians that treat these infants. As far as we are aware, there has never been another treatment proven to be as effective for treating colic as chiropractic!

One of the most dramatic cases that we ever witnessed was with an infant with colic. This case was actually the younger sister of KB who was one of the case studies in Chapter Five who had apnea. LB was a very fussy baby. She did not sleep or eat well and cried almost constantly for two weeks. Her mother brought her in to have her atlas examined at The Sweat Chiropractic Clinic for Atlas Orthogonality at two weeks of age. After approximately two hours in the office while she was examined and x-rayed following the Atlas Orthogonal Procedure, we began to understand how a tired, frustrated parent might loose their temper with the constant crying of a colicky infant. While Dr. Craig (the co-author of this book) was attending to another patient, Dr. Tracey (co-author) was assisting in the adjusting of LB. Immediately after the adjustment, the baby stopped crying and fell asleep. The results were so dramatic, it was difficult to believe it was the same child. When Dr. Craig saw the infant sleeping in the mother's arms, he said, "Is that the same baby?" She was hardly recognizable since before the adjustment her face was red from the constant crying, and now she was a peaceful, sleeping baby with normal color.

Another case of colic responding well to atlas adjusting comes from Dr. Mitch Aumont in Sainte-Croix, Quebec, Canada. Audrey was born to a healthy twenty-nine year old woman. The birth was a vaginal delivery with no remarkable or complicating factors. Audrey had good Apgar scores (nine and ten), but did not breast-feed right away. At fifteen days of age, Audrey developed colic, which consisted of crying every three hours for at least an hour, she did not eat at all and had a very difficult time sleeping. At twenty days old, when the mother brought Audrey in to see Dr. Aumont she asked, "Can you please help my baby, because I had another baby that had the same symptoms and she died?"

After an examination revealed that Audrey had an atlas subluxation, she was given an Atlas Orthogonal adjustment. After one adjustment the symptoms cleared up almost immediately. Audrey was examined on five other office visits, but was in adjustment. No further treatment was required and her symptoms never returned.

It may be difficult for some people to understand how this procedure can be effective with symptoms such as colic. We too are often amazed with some of the results achieved with atlas adjusting. The research that we found while writing this book has helped to make it more clear how the atlas adjustment can be such a powerful tool in treating many symptoms and disorders and improving overall health. The brain stem and the rest of the nerve system control all functions in the body. When the nerves and blood vessels become free of pressure and irritation, the body is able to work in a more normal manner, improving many aspects of health.

Can Chiropractic Improve Breast Feeding?

Recently one of our medical colleagues suggested to us that if we can show that chiropractic can improve brain stem function, then a conclusion could be drawn that since suckling is dependent on the brain stem, then breast feeding may be improved upon following infant adjusting. Since hungry babies become fussy babies, this connection may be another way that chiropractic can help to reduce colic and protect infants from shaken baby syndrome.

Accidents: The Leading Cause of Death in Children

As a side note here, we would like to remind people that childhood accidents are the leading cause of death in children ages 1–14 years old. A study of 536 infants conducted by the National Safety Council discovered that 255 (47.5%) had fallen from a high place during the first year of life. This can occur simply by leaving an infant unattended while on a changing table, couch or bed, even for just a few seconds.

A 1990 study from the U.S. Consumer Product Safety Commissioner revealed that almost a quarter of a million children under the age of fifteen were treated for injuries related to playground equipment. The majority of these accidents were falls, with approximately 50% resulting in head and neck trauma. If deaths from accidents and severe trauma are so common, how many children survive accidents, slips and falls (from changing tables, bunk beds, bicycles, skateboards, roller skates, swing sets, tree forts, etc.), and go through life subluxated? Very frequently, a trauma or fall will precede some type of symptom in a pediatric patient. We see this pattern when performing case histories. It only stands to reason that children should regularly be examined by a chiropractor.

We don't want to make parents paranoid, however, we must be aware of the potential spinal damage that can take place when accidents happen. We all need to be diligent in taking precautions to reduce and avoid potential accidents. Parents also need to be aware that if and when their child does have some sort of trauma (which is often unavoidable) they need to have their necks examined by their chiropractor. Too often these silent yet damaging spinal subluxations go undetected and may have serious long-term health consequences.

7

Infant Wellness Review and Steps to SIDS Prevention

Medical and scientific researchers have identified malfunction of the brain stem as the area most likely to be the cause leading to SIDS in many cases.

Chiropractic care, focusing on the upper cervical spine, specifically the atlas, may be able to reduce the damaging effects of the vertebral subluxation complex (VSC) and may be able to improve abnormal brain stem function. Whether cramped by uterine or abdominal constraints before the birth process begins, or by being twisted and stretched in the trip through the birth canal, many newborns have misalignments in their necks, which cause nerve interference. Our research suggests that this interference can lead to SIDS, or at the very least, to sub-optimum health conditions as the child develops. It is imperative that all infants have their atlas examined by a chiropractor shortly after birth. This is especially urgent if there were any complications during the pregnancy, labor or delivery, or if the infant has respiratory abnormalities or other type of symptom.

Chiropractic has been shown to be effective for many childhood diseases and symptoms. One of the most promising studies on chiropractic and infantile colic was published in 1999 and showed that chiropractic can reduce infantile colic by nearly 75%. Chiropractic has also been cited as effective in treating seizures, bed-wetting, and ear infections. It is time the general public knows the wonderful health benefits of chiropractic.

Pregnancy and Birth Options

We would like to offer a few suggestions on how to deliver healthier babies. One is to have the mother receive regular chiropractic care during the pregnancy. Several studies have been published that show the effectiveness of chiropractic care for pregnant women. One study demonstrated that 75% of pregnant women responded favorably to chiropractic care in regards to symptoms, primarily low back pain.[1]

Another study worth mentioning shows promise regarding the effectiveness of chiropractic on reducing the time a pregnant woman is in labor. Dr. Joan Fallon reported that in pregnant woman under chiropractic care, labor was reduced by 25% in first pregnancies and by 31% in subsequent pregnancies.[2] Since many authorities believe the major source of trauma sustained by an infant during the birth process is the actual labor, treating pregnant women and reducing the amount of time they are in labor may be an important step in delivering healthier infants.

In general, we recommend that the fewer interventions a woman receives while in labor and delivery, the better, this includes the use of any drugs. A paper written by three Danish doctors and published in 1991 supports this statement. They reported that when a woman's labor was induced because the doctor was concerned that the fetus was getting too large, several negative results occurred compared to woman that were allowed to go into spontaneous labor with the same sized fetus. These results included:

- The frequency of emergency cesarean section surgery was tripled.

- The frequency of vacuum extraction was doubled.

- Significantly more infants had Apgar scores of less than 7 after one minute. The Apgar score is method of assessing an infant at birth. The Apgar score measures five health components: appearance (color), pulse rate, grimace (facial response), activity (muscle tone), and respiratory effort. A score under seven means the baby needs some level of additional help.

The authors stated:

It is concluded that induction of labour is not indicated in cases where a large fetus is suspected.[3]

Another paper that supports the natural approach to labor and delivery was published in 1993 in The American Journal of Obstetrics and Gynecology.[4] The study reported that when a baby was delivered by a certified nurse-midwife, the following results occurred:

- The chance of having a cesarean section was significantly reduced.

- There was a lower risk of abnormal labor.

- There was a lower incidence of fetal distress, producing healthier infants.

The authors stated:

This work demonstrates that labor abnormalities and diagnosis of fetal distress are less frequent in patients cared for by nurse-midwives, and there is an association with a lower incidence of cesarean section.

Caution in using drugs in childbirth

Mothers-to-be need to understand the effects of epidurals and other pain killing drugs given during labor of which most are narcotic drugs. One of the effects of narcotics is respiratory depression. Another reason to avoid such drugs is because the mother is unable to work with her body and push the baby out effectively as she can no longer feel her contractions. Therefore, she must rely on machines and technology to tell her when to push. This may lead to other more serious interventions, which may cause more complications. As evidence to this statement, an article published in *The American Journal of Obstetrics and Gynecology* found that epidurals were associated with an increased need of the use of forceps in the delivery of the baby.[5] Several articles have also been published on the complications associated with epidurals.[6–10] These complications include:

- Increased time the mother is in labor.
- Increased risk of fever for the mother and baby.
- Increased risk of antibiotics given to the newborn.
- Increased risk of seizures in the baby.
- Risk of paralysis for the mother.
- Risk of puncture of the spinal cord.

We recommend that parents-to-be become as educated as possible about the entire birth process, from pregnancy to delivery. The American Academy of Husband-Coached Childbirth (The Bradley Method) is a great resource for education and preparing for the new baby. They can be reached at (800) 42-BIRTH.

According to the Bradley Method:

The kind of pregnancy, labor and delivery our children experience has a profound and lifelong effect on their health, including their mental and emotional health. On many issues (or interventions), even experts cannot agree. This places the challenge of decision making directly on the parents' shoulders. Knowing the issues, and the pros and cons, can make a difference.

They also recommend:

Make a realistic birth plan to encourage you to have good communications with your birth team so you can work together toward the goal of the safest and most positive experience possible. For the majority of well-trained women, allowing labor to follow the natural course is the best and safest route. Medications and other interventions, such as cesarean sections, may be life saving in specific circumstances, but always have their own special additional risks. Labors should be evaluated on an individual basis, not routine. Machines cannot replace good personal care.[11]

As well as recommending good nutrition, exercising regularly, and relaxation to reduce and handle the pain you experience, the Bradley Method warns against the dangerous effects of epidurals. They stated:

The American Academy of Pediatrics, Committee on Drugs has stated that there

*is no drug either by prescription, over-the-counter or food additive that has
ever been proven safe for the unborn baby. All childbirth pain medications,
"relaxers", and anesthetics do reach the unborn baby, usually within one
minute.*[11]

We also feel the need to mention the fact that ultrasound is non-ionizing radiation
and very few studies have been performed on the safety of this test on fetuses. Many
parents, not knowing this is radiation, gladly have this test performed nearly on every
prenatal visit. We want to call people's attention to this and ask to see the research on
the safety of this test and the long-term effects on baby's health. This means any-
time the nurse, doctor or mid-wife wants to put gel on your abdomen to hear the
baby's heart beat, they are about to use ultrasound. It takes a little more skill, but in
most cases, a feta-scope can be used just as well to hear the baby's heart beat. In some
cases, ultrasound may be necessary but should be reserved for the high-risk cases
since ultrasound's long-term effects have not been determined.

It is not our intention to scare a pregnant mother, however we feel it is important to
advise mothers-to-be of the many risks associated with interventions during birth.
From the above referenced articles it is clear to see that a safer birth may be achieved
through avoiding drugs in labor. One typical reply we hear when we warn of drugs
in labor is, "I used drugs during my labor and my kids are fine." We want to know,
"They are fine compared to what? And how much better could they be if the drugs
had been avoided?" Just knowing the risks associated with the drugs and procedures
should make a pregnant woman want to avoid them. If you can avoid it, why put
your newborn who is so vulnerable at risk at all?

Recommendations for the parents-to-be and parents of a newborn

(For the sake of ease in reading this section, we refer to the infant as a baby boy).

1. Talk to your OBGYN, midwives, or the team that will be assisting in the delivery
    of your baby. Ask them to take extra precaution with your newborn's head and
    neck as he is being delivered and as the team assists in the process of cleaning,
    measuring, weighing and other procedures done to the infant upon delivery.
    Think about the miracle that has just taken place: this fetus was growing inside
    the mother and now has presented itself to the world. Try to make his entrance
    as peaceful as possible. In our opinion, as a general rule, the less intervention the
    better when it comes to childbirth and delivery.

2. When you handle your new baby and when you allow others to handle him, treat
    the entire body as one unit, keeping your infant's head and neck in line with the
    rest of his body. Do not allow his head to flop or be tilted to one side at all. When
    bathing especially, take extreme care in the handling of his head and neck.

3. Please do not bounce your baby or even gently toss him up and down. This can
    create micro-trauma in the infant's spine and usually subluxates an infant. Make
    sure you also stress this to relatives (aunts and uncles are notorious "bouncers"
    and "tossers"), as well as to baby-sitters, especially teenage baby-sitters.

4. Car seats and strollers are another common cause of spinal misalignments. When
    we walk through a mall we frequently see someone pushing a sleeping infant in

a stroller with the infant's head tilted over to one side, with the ear almost touching the shoulder. Can this be good for an infant's spine? Of course not! So please, make sure you have a rolled up towel or infant pillow so that you can support your baby's head when he is in a car seat or stroller. We should mention that this special attention should not end when the child becomes a toddler or older. Whenever you or your child fall asleep, make sure the head and neck are not in a compromised position. It is a good idea to always carry a small pillow in the car in case your child falls asleep, so he can have support to his head and neck.

5. When your baby becomes mobile (starts to crawl and eventually walk) always keep a gate in front of any stairs. Children have a tendency to be drawn towards stairs and it only takes a second or two for there to be a major accident.

6. Have your child's atlas examined shortly after birth, or any trauma or fall to ensure proper spinal alignment, which can lead to a healthier childhood. As a side note here, we want to point out the fact that after a small child falls down or is injured, the first thing that people do is check the child for any bleeding. We assume that if he is not bleeding than he must be all right. Again this is an area that awareness needs to be raised as falls and minor traumas are frequent causes of spinal misalignment, and can have long-term health consequences.

The following suggestions may increase an infant's health and help reduce the risk of SIDS:

- Early and regular prenatal care provides a healthy start for any baby.

- Proper nutrition for the pregnant mother should include a focus on protein, natural healthy foods and folic acid.

- Avoid taking any unnecessary drugs.

- Pregnant women should exercise and receive chiropractic care.

- Place your baby on its back or side to sleep. This recommendation from the American Academy of Pediatrics and the National Back to Sleep Campaign applies to most babies. Since some babies seem to insist on sleeping on their stomachs, it is a good idea to have something to prevent them from rolling onto their stomachs, such as a rolled up towel or firm cylinder pillow. Place this pillow snug up to the baby from the level of his arms down, to prevent him from rolling over. This helps to ensure that he will not be twisting his neck, which may compromise the important nerve structures in this area.

- Don't smoke; provide a smoke-free environment for babies in your care and encourage parents who smoke to quit. Recent research indicates that the risk of SIDS doubles among babies exposed only after birth to cigarette smoke and triples for those exposed both during pregnancy and after birth. Infants exposed to smoke also have more colds and other upper respiratory tract infections.

- Breastfeed your baby. Studies show that babies who died of SIDS were less likely to have been breastfed. Breast-feeding is important since breast milk contains antibodies and nutrients that can prevent gastrointestinal and respiratory illnesses and infections.

- Do not keep small objects or stuffed toys in the crib with your baby, as these items may cause choking.

- Change your baby on the floor instead of a couch, bed or changing table that he may fall off of (this will also decrease the stress on your back).

- When you are changing the baby, be sure not to lift his feet or bottom too high, as this may put unnecessary stress on the infant's neck and upper back.

- Use a firm, flat mattress in a safety-approved crib. The U.S. Consumer Product Safety Commission has issued advisories for parents on the hazards to infants sleeping on beanbag cushions, sheepskins, foam pads, foam sofa cushions, synthetic-filled adult pillows, and foam pads covered with comforters, as these products may inhibit breathing.

- Under certain circumstances, certain adult bedding may pose a threat to infants, so exercise extreme caution if your baby sleeps in your bed with you.

- Educate other potential caregivers to your baby, such as baby-sitters, daycare workers, friends and grandparents on the importance of spinal care. Do not assume they know even the basic safety precautions.

- Learn Infant CPR.

- Have your baby checked for vertebral subluxations, especially at the level of the atlas, as soon as possible after birth.

If a child in your care is not breathing and is unresponsive:

- Immediately notify emergency medical personnel (dial 911).

- Begin cardiopulmonary resuscitation (CPR).

We must keep in mind the sad truth that any baby may be vulnerable to SIDS despite his parents' best efforts to prevent it. Therefore, it is imperative that we all continue to support scientific research and that we keep open minds to new and alternative approaches. Only in this manner will we uncover other risk factors, possible causes, and treatments that may offer solutions to the SIDS puzzle.

8

StopSIDS.org

StopSIDS.org is a non-profit organization dedicated to research and education to end sudden infant death syndrome (SIDS) and other senseless infant deaths. Our goal is to promote optimum health in babies and children through chiropractic-atlas correction and other healthy lifestyle choices. It is a "health hub" for research, fundraising, and communications about SIDS and its prevention, as well as improved infant and child health.

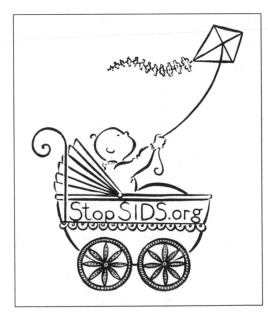

The StopSIDS.org *logo was drawn by Shawn Banner. It is a whimsical representation of a healthy baby. The kite, with the spine as its tail encompasses the philosophy for the organization, which incorporates:*

1. *Taking Flight*
2. *Soaring to New Heights*
3. *The Sky's The Limit*

It represents the belief that true health and a child's full potential can only be achieved with a properly functioning nerve system, which can be obtained through chiropractic care.

What we hope to accomplish through writing this book and the efforts of the non-profit organization ***StopSIDS.org***, is to educate the public that a correlation exists between the atlas vertebral subluxation complex, the atlas neuro-vascular syndrome and SIDS. We plan on performing research studies on infants who have been identified as being "at risk" for SIDS, or "near-miss SIDS cases" to show that the atlas adjustment can have positive effects on these cases and can improve abnormal brain stem function. We have set up an international research project involving doctors across the United States, Canada, Japan and Australia. The results of the project will be updated on our Web site (www.*StopSIDS.org*) and when completed, published in a scientific journal. If the results of the research show positive improvement in brain stem function and improved respiratory and cardiac function, we believe one of the major pieces to the SIDS puzzle will have been solved—a bold statement, but one we truly believe!

As you have seen from many of the research papers that have been published, chiropractic care can have a dramatic impact on children's health. The challenge we have with SIDS and doing research to suggest a preventative value from chiropractic treatment is that SIDS is a diagnosis that is only made after the death of an infant, and it is nearly impossible to "prove prevention." Much of the medical research suggests the brain stem is associated with SIDS. We have seen children's health, particularly difficulty in breathing normalize after specific atlas adjusting. It is our hope that the research studies planned through *StopSIDS.org* will prove the important connection between adjusting the atlas vertebra and improved infant health. From that knowledge we hope to draw the conclusion that children under chiropractic care are less likely to succumb to SIDS.

In a recently published paper by Dr. Dale Mortenson, he stated that he has asked many chiropractors if they have ever had an infant that they were treating die of SIDS. The answer has always been "No." He stated,

> *According to most upper cervical theories, the evidence points to a misalignment of C-1, creating pressure or distortion of the lower medulla and causing disruption of the normal neural transmission in this region. It would stand to reason that upper cervical chiropractors have the answer in their hands to sudden infant death syndrome. We therefore have an obligation to check as many children as possible for atlas subluxation and adjust when necessary.*[1]

Important research has been performed to date that points to the brain stem and abnormal respiratory control in the cause of SIDS. Medical doctors are so close to the problem but they must understand how powerful an atlas adjustment is and recognize its possible link to SIDS and improving infant health. Some of the most exciting research has come from Dr. Hanna Kinney at Children's Hospital in Boston, with her focus on the brain stem. She and her research team have identified the area of the brain stem that frequently shows abnormalities in SIDS victims. Doctors at the University of California at Los Angeles (UCLA) have found abnormal respiratory control in infants who later died of SIDS. It is difficult to control our emotions as we realize how close they are to understanding the problem. We must be vigilant in our research efforts and raise the awareness that the problem may very well lie in the alignment of the upper cervical spine. Children are dying every day, needless drugs are being taken, and surgeries are being performed due to the fact that parents are unaware that their infants could have a misalignment in their upper neck that could be life-threatening.

In order to achieve optimum health, every baby needs to have a healthy spinal column. It is the framework that will support a child throughout his or her growing years and adulthood. Studies have shown that newborn infants often enter the world with spinal trauma due to malposition in the womb and the stress of the birth process. Even under the best conditions, birthing can be traumatic for the infant, who has spent nine months cradled in the dark, warm comfort of the womb. It is very important to have your infant's upper neck examined by a chiropractor shortly after his or her birth to be certain that there is no nerve interference. Periodic checks should continue throughout your child's lifetime.

We look forward to the day when neck examinations of infants are on the same plane that vaccinations are today – mandatory in most cases. If it can be mandated that toxins be injected into our children's bodies, then why can't a vital, health improving modality such as upper cervical chiropractic care be mandated? We understand this idea is ahead of its time, but we also understand that public opinion is not the same thing as truth or fact or always in the best interest of health.

Your help is needed today! Please buy this book for your friends and family members, especially if they are expecting a baby or are already parents of a child. Buy a copy of this book for your medical doctor, and any pediatricians in your area, remember a portion of every sale goes directly towards infant research projects. Visit the *www.StopSIDS.org* site and make a tax-deductible donation today. With your help, we will be able to make great strides in further researching SIDS, developing an effective campaign for its prevention and improving infant health which will have a dramatic long term positive impact on the human health potential.

About the Authors

Dr. Craig Wehrenberg and Dr. Tracey Mulhall-Wehrenberg are Board Certified Atlas Orthogonal Chiropractors. They have been in private practice in upstate New York since 1992. They are graduates of Life Chiropractic College in Marietta, Georgia. They began studying the Atlas Orthogonal Procedure in 1988 while they were Research Assistants at Life, where they became extremely impressed with the improved health results obtained through atlas correction. In their experience, they have seen many different types of cases improve with Atlas Orthogonal chiropractic. Some of these cases include infant apnea, infant colic, cerebral palsy, seizure disorders, hypertension and hyperactivity.

Through the non-profit organization StopSIDS.org, the doctors hope to perform research and educate the public on the importance of atlas adjusting and its relationship to SIDS and improved infant health.

Glossary

Adjustment—A correction of a spinal subluxation (misalignment) in order to reduce it and restore normal nerve function.

Atlantal-occipital—The connection between the atlas (C1) and the bone at the base of the head called the occiput.

Atlas (C1)—The first cervical vertebra.

Atlas Neuro-Vascular Syndrome (ANVS)—The condition when an atlas vertebral subluxation causes nerve and vascular compromise, affecting functions throughout the body. Associated with this syndrome is mechanical spinal cord and brain stem deformation. There may also be dysfunction of the neuroanatomy in the brain and brain stem through the complex feedback mechanisms of the joints in the upper neck, as well as loss of normal blood supply to the brain stem through the vertebral arteries and other vascular structures in this area.

Atlas Orthogonal Chiropractic—Atlas Orthogonality (pronounced or thog' ah nality) is chiropractic program designed to find and correct spinal subluxations based on scientific and biomechanical procedures. It is a system to reduce neurological insult by balancing anatomical structures, primarily the atlas vertebra without the use of manual manipulation. It incorporates the use of a state-of-the-art floor-based percussion adjusting instrument and precision x-ray analysis. A board-certified Atlas Orthogonist is a doctor of chiropractic that is recognized as a specialist in the field of chiropractic, with advanced training in the structure, function, and biomechanics of the upper cervical spine, specifically the atlas. Dr. Roy Sweat of Atlanta, Georgia developed the Atlas Orthogonal procedure, the adjusting and x-ray instruments.

Autonomic Nerve System—The part of the nervous system that controls all automatic functions such as organ and glandular function.

Axis (C2)—The second cervical vertebra.

Brain stem—The area of the central nervous system that connects the brain to the spinal cord and consists of nervous tissue essential for the existence of life.

Chiropractic—First developed in 1895, today chiropractic is the largest drugless healing profession. Chiropractic is based on the scientific fact that the nerve system controls the function of every cell, tissue, organ and system in your body. The nerve system consists of the brain, spinal cord and millions of nerves. The brain is protected by the skull, and the spinal cord is protected by the 24 movable bones of the spine. Many everyday activities can cause these spinal bones to lose their normal position. This can result in nervous system dysfunction and ultimately ill health. The chiropractic approach to better health is to detect, reduce and help prevent nervous system dysfunction.

Foramen Magnum—The opening at the base of the skull, which the spinal cord descends through. This level is considered by many to be the junction of the spinal column and the brain stem.

Histopathology—Abnormal soft tissue function.

Myopathology—Abnormal muscle function.

Neuropathophysiology—Abnormal nervous system function.

Occiput—The base of the skull bone which articulates with the atlas (the first cervical vertebra).

Orthogonal—To be at right angles

Pathophysiology—Abnormal function of the spine and body.

Spinal Kinesiopathology—Abnormal motion or position of spinal bones.

Subluxation—A bone of the spine that is out of its proper position, causing nerve interference.

The Atlas VSC-SIDS Theory—A theory that incorporates the relationship between the first bone in the spine (C1, also known as the atlas) and the critical neurological and vascular structures that affect cardiac and respiratory function, that are located in this area, as a cause of SIDS. This theory recognizes that there may be other causes of SIDS, and this is presented as one theory.

When an atlas (the first vertebra in the spine) becomes subluxated in an infant the following can take place:

- Abnormal spinal cord and brain stem function due to direct mechanical stretching of these structures.

- Electrical and chemical signals to and from the brain become disturbed.

- A decrease in the proper blood supply to the brain stem from the vertebral arteries which may be altered due to the malposition of the atlas.

Due to the fact that the infant nerve system and brain stem are not fully matured, infants are at particular risk of serious health consequences from nerve system insult.

Upper Cervical Spine—The upper neck. Typically the occiput, Atlas (C-1), and Axis (C-2) are included in this term.

Vagus Nerve—The tenth cranial nerve, which originates in the brain stem and affects many areas such as the heart, lungs, stomach, ears, pharynx, larynx, trachea, esophagus, the majority of the autonomic functions and internal organs

Vertebra—A bone in the spine that, with 23 other vertebrae, the sacrum and coccyx makes up the vertebral or spinal column. The vertebral column houses and protects the spinal cord.

Vertebral Arteries—Blood vessels that pass through openings in the neck vertebrae from C-6 to C-1, and supply one-third to one-half of the blood to the brain including the brain stem, cerebellum, and parts of the cerebrum.

Vertebral Subluxation Complex (VSC)—A misalignment of a vertebra in the spine causing nerve interference, and five components:

1. *Spinal Kinesiopathology*—Abnormal spinal movement
2. *Neuropathophysiology*—Abnormal nerve function
3. *Myopathology*—Abnormal muscle function
4. *Histopathology*—Abnormal cellular changes
5. *Pathophysiology*—Spinal and systemic degeneration and disorders

Zygapophyseal joints—The joints that connect each vertebra to the one above and below it.

References

CHAPTER ONE

1. Dunne KB, Clarren SK. "The origin of prenatal and postnatal deformities." Pediatr Clin North Am. 1986 Dec; 33(6):1277–97.

2. Flesia JM. "The vertebral subluxation complex part III-pathogenesis." *International Review of Chiropractic* Nov/Dec 1992; 45–47.

3. Webster L. "Subluxation at Birth and Early Childhood." International *Chiropractic Pediatric Association*, March 1989.

4. Fysh PN. "Clinical Implications of Birth Trauma to the Brainstem and Upper Cervical Spine in Newborn Infants." Proceedings from International Chiropractors Association Scientific Research Symposium, Tampa, Fla., 1990.

5. Yates P. "Birth Trauma to the Vertebral Arteries." *Arch Dis Child* 34:436, 1959.

6. Gould SJ, Smith JF. "Spinal cord transection, cerebral ischaemic and brain-stem injury in a baby following a Kielland's forceps rotation." *Neuropathol Appl Neurobiol* 1984 Mar-Apr;10(2):151–8.

7. Pridmore BR, Aherne WA. "Spinal cord injury of the fetus during delivery with Kielland's forceps." *J Obstet Gynaecol Br Commonw* 1974 Feb;81(2):168–72.

8. Pridmore BR, Aherne WA. "Spinal cord injury of the fetus during delivery with Kielland's forceps." *J Obstet Gynaecol Br Commonw* 1974 Feb;81(2):168–72.

9. Craig S, McClure G. "A preterm infant with upper cervical spinal cord injury, following delivery with Kielland's forceps." *J Perinat Med* 1997;25(6):502–4.

10. Menticoglou SM, Perlman M, Manning FA. "High cervical spinal cord injury in neonates delivered with forceps: report of 15 cases." *Obstet Gynecol* 1995 Oct;86(4 Pt 1):589–94.

11. Healy DL. "Design errors in Kielland's forceps." *Aust N Z J Obstet Gynaecol* 1982 Feb;22(1):31–3.

12. Cruikshank DP. "High cervical spinal cord injury in neonates delivered with forceps: report of 15 cases." *Obstet Gynecol* 1996 Feb;87(2):319–20.

13. Nuijen S, Hausman R. "Fatal forceps." *Med Sci Law* 1983 Oct;23(4):254–6.

14. Finch J. "A complicated case: brain damage caused by forceps delivery." *Nurs Mirror* 1981 Jan 8;152(2):7.

15. Pamphlett R, Cala A. "Spinal cord injury after forceps rotation: the role of glioneuronal heterotopias." *Aust N Z J Obstet Gynaecol* 1993 Feb;33(1):91–3.

16. Ruggieri M, Smarason AK, Pike M. "Spinal cord insults in the prenatal, perinatal, and neonatal periods." *Dev Med Child Neurol* 1999 May; 41(5):311–7.

17. Shaver DC, Bada HS, Korones SB, Anderson GD, Wong SP, Arheart KL. "Early and

late intraventricular hemorrhage: the role of obstetric factors." *Obstet Gynecol* 1992 Nov;80 (5):831–7.

18. Plauche WC. "Fetal cranial injuries related to delivery with the Malmstrom vacuum extractor." *Obstet Gynecol* 1979 Jun;53(6):750–7.

19. O'Leary JA, Ferrell RE, Randolph CR. "Retinal hemorrhage and vacuum extraction delivery." *J Perinat Med* 1986;14(3):197–9.

20. Seidman DS, Laor A, Gale R, Stevenson DK, Mashiach S, Danon YL. "Long-term effects of vacuum and forceps deliveries." *Lancet* 1991 Jun 29; 337(8757):1583–5.

21. Naske R, Poustka F, Presslich O, Schubert H, Zapotoczky HG, Altmann P, Schaller A. "[Connectons between instrumental delivery and cerebral damage in the infant]." *Wien Klin Wochenschr* 1976 May 14;88(10):319–24.

22. Krause W, Frenzel J, Raphael M, Michels W. "Significance of trial vacuum extraction in the framework of obstetric surgery in vertex presentation." *Geburtshilfe Frauenheilkd* 1985 Aug;45(8):539–45.

23. Plauche WC. Subgaleal hematoma. "A complication of instrumental delivery." *Ugeskr Laeger* 1991 Jan 14;153(3):181–3.

24. Wangala P, Riethmuller D, Nguyen S, Maillet R, Colette C. "Unrecognized hemorrhages during delivery." *Rev Fr Gynecol Obstet* 1995 Apr-May;90(4):215–9.

25. Dierker LJ Jr, Rosen MG, Thompson K, Debanne S, Linn P. "The midforceps: maternal and neonatal outcomes." *Am J Obstet Gynecol* 1985 May 15;152(2):176–83.

26. Galbraith RS. "Incidence of neonatal sixth nerve palsy in relation to mode of delivery." *Am J Obstet Gynecol* 1994 Apr;170(4):1158–9.

27. Towner D, Castro MA, Eby-Wilkens E, "Gilbert WM. Effect of mode of delivery in nulliparous women on neonatal intracranial injury." *N Engl J Med* 1999 Dec 2;341(23):1709–14.

28. Vacca A. Correspondence: N Engl J Med. 2000 Mar 23 ;342 (12).

29. DiMarco CS, Ramsey PS, Williams LH, Ramin KD. "Temporal trends in operative obstetric delivery: 1992–1999." *Obstet Gynecol* 2000 Apr 1;95(4 Suppl 1):S39)

30. Holden KR, Titus MO, Van Tassel P. "Cranial magnetic resonance imaging examination of normal term neonates: a pilot study." *J Child Neurol* 1999 Nov;14(11):708–10.

31. Abroms I. "Cervical Cord Injuries Secondary to Hyperextension of the Head in Breech Presentations." Obstet Gynecol 41:369, 1973.

32. Painter MD, Depp R, O'Donoghue P. "Fetal Heart Rate Patterns and Development in the first year of life." Am Obstet Gynecol 132:271, 1978.

33. The Peter Pan Potential Seminars. The Peter Pan Potential. 4201 N. Clovis Avenue Fresno, CA.

34. Towbin A. "Latent spinal cord and brain stem injury in newborn infants." Develop Med Child Neurol. 1969 Feb; 11 (1): 54–68.

35. Towbin A. "Spinal Cord and Brainstem Injury at Birth." Arch Path 1964, 77: 620.

36. Morley R, Kennedy K, Lucas A, Blizzard L, Dwyer T. "Mode of delivery and childhood blood pressure." *Pediatr Res* 2000 Apr;47(4 Pt 1):463–7.

37. Frazier JP, Cleary TG, Pickering LK, Kohl S, Ross PJ. "Leukocyte function in healthy neonates following vaginal and cesarean section deliveries." *J Pediatr* 1982 Aug;101(2):269–72

38. Bowers SK, MacDonald HM, Shapiro ED. "Prevention of iatrogenic neonatal

respiratory distress syndrome: elective repeat cesarean section and spontaneous labor." *Am J Obstet Gynecol* 1982 May 15;143(2):186–9.

39. Gilles FH, Bina M, Sotrel A. "Infantile Atlanto-occipital Instability: The Potential Danger of Extreme Extension." Am J Dis Child 1979; Vol 133: pp30–7.

40. Hospers LA, et al. "Atlanto-Occipital Hypermobility in Sudden Infant Death Syndrome." Today's Chiropractic Jan/Feb, 1990; 19 (1): 36–40.

41. Rossitch E Jr, Oakes WJ. "Perinatal spinal cord injury: Clinical, radiographic and pathologic features." *Pediatr Neurosurg* 1992; 18(3): 149–52.

42. Biedermann H. "Kinematic Imbalances due to Suboccipital strain in newborns," *Medicine* Springer-Verlag 1992, 151–156.

42. Gutmann G. "Blocked Atlantal Nerve Syndrome in Infants and Small Children." Originally published in *Manuelle Medizine*, Springer-Verlag, 1987. English translation published in *International Review of Chiropractic* July/Aug 1990; 37–43.

CHAPTER TWO

1. Palmer BJ. Chiropractic Clinical Controlled Research. WB Conkey Company, Hamond, Indiana, 1951.

2. Grostic JD. "Somatosensory evoked potentials in chiropractic research." *Today's Chiropractic* 21(3): 56–58, 1990.

3. Grostic JD, Glick DM, Burke E, Sheres B. "Chiropractic Adjustment Reversal of neurological insult: A preliminary report." Foundation for Chiropractic Education and Research, International Conference on Spinal Manipulation Proceedings, 1992.

4. Glick DM, Lee F. "Differential Diagnostic Somatosensory Evoked Potentials." *Chiro Research Journal* 2(2): 38–47, 1992.

5. Kent C, Gentempo P. "Paraspinal EMG Scanning in Chiropractic Practice: A Review." *Chiro Research Journal* 2(1): 41–49, 1991.

6. Dorland's Med Dictionary: 28th ed. Philadelphia : Saunders.

7. McMullen M. "Physical Stresses of Childhood that Could Lead to the Need for Chiropractic Care." *Proceedings of the National Conference on Chiropractic and Pediatrics*, San Diego, California. Int Chiropractors Assoc. 1991.

8. Walton EV. "The effects of chiropractic treatment on students with learning and behavior impairments due to neurological dysfunction. *Int. Rev Chiro* 1975; 29:4–5, 24–6.

9. Giesen JM, Center DB, Leach RA. "An evaluation of chiropractic manipulation as a treatment of hyperactivity in children." *J Manipulative Physiol Ther* 1989; 12(5): 353–63.

10. Hospers LA, Fiorini D, Tejada M, Mulhall TE, Wehrenberg CR. "Electroencephalographic Observations of Children with Petit Mal and Petit Mal/Grand Mal Variant Epilepsies Before and After Life Upper Cervical Adjustment." *Proceedings from International Chiropractors Association Scientific Research Symposium,* Tampa, Fla., 1990.

11. Gutmann G. "Blocked Atlantal Nerve Syndrome in Infants and Small Children." Originally published in Manuelle Medizine, Springer-Verlag, 1987. English translation published in *International Review of Chiropractic* July/Aug 1990; 37–43.

12. Hospers LA, Daso JA, Steinle LV. "Electromyographic Patterns of Mentally Retarded Cerebral Palsy Patient after Life Upper Cervical Adjustment." *Today's Chiropractic*, 15(5),13–14,1986.

13. Hospers LA, Sweat RW, LaRee H, Trotta N, Sweat MH. "Response of a Three-Year-Old Epileptic Child to Upper Cervical Adjustment." *Today's Chiropractic*, 15(15) 69–76, Dec–Jan 1987.

14. Goodman RJ, Mosby JS. "Cessation of a Seizure Disorder: Correction of the Atlas Subluxation Complex." *The Journal of Chiropractic Research and Clinical Investigation*,6(2), 43–46,1990.

15. Young G. "Chiropractic Success in Epileptic Conditions." *ACA Journal of Chiropractic* 1982; 19(4):62–63.

16. Hendricks CL, Larkin -Thier SM. "Otitis Media in Young Children." *Chiropractic* Jan. 1989 2(1); 9–13.

17. Froehle RM. "Ear infection: a retrospective study examining improvement from chiropractic care and analyzing for influencing factors." *J Manipulative Physiol Ther* 1996 Mar;19 (3): 169–177.

18. Fysh, PN. "Chronic Recurrent Otitis Media: Case Series of Five Patients With Recommendations for Case Management." *J of Clin Chiro Pediatrics.* 1996. 1(2). 66.

19. Vanbreda WM, Vanbreda J. "A Comparative Study of Health Status of Children Raised Under the Health Care Models of Chiropractic & Allopathic Medicine" *The American Chiropractor*, September 1993.

20. Gilman G, Bergstrand J. "Visual Recovery Following Chiropractic Intervention." *Journal of Behavioral Optometry* 1990 1(3); 73–74.

21. Stephens D, Pollard H, Bilton D, Thomson P, Gorman F. "Bilateral simultaneous optic nerve dysfunction after periorbital trauma: recovery of vision in association with with chiropractic spinal manipulation therapy." *J Manipulative Physiol Ther* 1999 Nov-Dec;22(9):615–21.

22. Korr IM: "Andrew Taylor Still memorial lecture: Research and Practice – a century later." *J Am Osteopathy Assoc* 1974 73:362.

23. Murray DR, Irwin M, Reardon CA, et al. "Sympathetic and immune interactions during dynamic exercise. Mediation via a beta 2 – adrenergic-dependent mechanism." *Circulation* 1992 86(1): 203.

24. Pero R. "Medical Researcher Excited By CBSRF Project Results." *The Chiropractic Journal*, August 1989; 32.

25. Brennan P, Graham M, Triano J, Hondras M. "Enhanced phagocytic cell respiratory bursts induced by spinal manipulation: Potential Role of Substance P." J Manip Physiolog Ther 1991; (14)7:399–400.

26. Selano JL, Hightower BC, Pfleger B, Feeley-Collins K, Grostic JD. "The Effects of Specific Upper Cervical Adjustments on the CD4 Counts of HIV Positive Patients." *The Chiro Research Journal*; 3(1); 1994.

27. Felton DL, Felton SY, Belonged DL, et al. "Noradrenergic sympathetic neural interactions with the immune system: structure and function." *Immunol Rev.* 1987 Dec;100:225–60.

28. Felton DL, Felton SY, Bellinger DL, Madden KS: "Fundamental aspects of neural-immune signaling." *Psy Psychosom.* 1993;60(1):46–56.)

29. Hossi J, Murphy GF, Egan CL, et al: "Regulation of Langerhorn cell function by nerves containing calcination gene-related peptide." *Nature* 1993 363(6425): 159.

30. Udem BJ: titled "Neural-immunologic interactions in asthma." *Hosp Pract* (Off Ed) 1994 29(2):59.

31. Sternberg EM, Chrousos GP, Wilder RI, Gold PW: "The stress responses and the regulation of inflammatory disease." *Ann Intern Med* 1992 117(10):854.

32. Fricchoine GL, Stefano GB: "The stress response and autoimmuno-regulation." *Adv Neuroimmunol* 1994 4(1):13.

33. Ottaway CA, Husband AJ: "Central nervous system influences on lymphocyte migration." *Brain Behav Immun* 1992 6(2):97.

34. Werhe E, Krekel J. "The neoroimmune connection in human tonsils." *Brain Behav Immun* 1991 5(1):41.

35. Brennan PC, Triano JJ, McGregor M, et al: "Enhanced neutrophil respiratory burst as a biological marker for manipulation forces:duration of the effect and association with substance P and tumor necrosis factor." *JMPT* 1992 15 (2):83.

36. Kent C. "Neuroimmunology and chiropractic." *The Chiropractic Journal* Oct 1995, 30–31.

37. Biedermann H. "Kinematic Imbalances due to Suboccipital strain in newborns." *Medicine* Springer-Verlag 1992, 151–156.

38. Koch LE, Biedermann H, Saternus KS. "High Cervical Stress and Apnoea." *Forensic Sci Int* 1998 Oct 12;97(1):1–9.

39. Windsor H. "Sympathetic segmental disturbances. The evidence of the association in dissected cadavers of visceral disease with vertebral deformities of the same sympathetic segments." Med Times 49:1–7, 1921.

CHAPTER THREE

1. Bergman A, Beckwith J, Ray C, et al. "Sudden Infant Death Syndrome." *Proceedings of the Second International Conference on the Causes of Sudden Death in infants.* Seattle: University of Washington Press, 1970: 14–22.

2. Willinger M, James LS, Catz C. "Defining the sudden infant death syndrome (SIDS): Deliberations of an expert panel convened by the National Institute of Child Health and Human Development." *Pediatr Pathol* 1991; 11:677–84.

3. Kinney HC, Filiano JJ, Harper RM. "The neuropathology of the sudden infant death syndrome. A review." *J Neuropathol Exp Neurol* 1992; 51:115–126.

4. The SIDS Alliance Web site, 1999

5. The SIDS Alliance. "Differentiating Between Sudden Infant Death Syndrome, Shaken Baby Syndrome, and Accidental Infant Deaths Associated With Bedsharing." Media Advisory, November 29, 1999

6. Table of SIDS Deaths and Mortality Rates per 1,000 Live Births for 1983 to 1997. National Sudden Infant Death Syndrome Resource Center, Vienna, VA, Sep 1999.

7. Gilbert-Barness E, Barness L. "Sudden Infant Death: A Reappraisal." *Contemp. Pediat* 12 (4):88–107, April 1995.

8. Mortenson D. "Sudden Infant Death Syndrome." *Vector* Spring 2000; 2(5): 11.

9. The National Sleep Foundation.

10. Schechtman VL, Lee MY, Wilson AJ, Harper RM. "Dynamics of respiratory patterning

in normal infants and infants who subsequently died of the sudden infant death syndrome." *Pediatr Res* 1992 Jun;31(6):606–12.

CHAPTER FOUR

1. Palmer DD. "The Chiropractic Adjuster." Portland, OR: *Portland Publishing Co,* 1910.

2. Crothers B. "Injury of Spinal Cord in breech extractions as important causes of fetal death and paraplegia in childhood." *Am J Med Sci;* 1923; 165:94.

3. Gilles FH, Dina M, Sorrel A. "Infantile Atlanto-occipital instability: the potential danger of extreme extension." *Am J Dis Child* 1979; 133:30–7.

4. Kinney HC, Filiano JJ, Harper RM. "The neuropathology of the sudden infant death syndrome. A review." *J Neuropathol Exp Neurol* 1992;51:115–126.

5. Filiano JJ, Kinney HC. "Arcuate Nucleus Hypoplasia in the Sudden Infant Death Syndrome." *J Neuropathol Exp Neurol* 1992;51:394–403.

6. Fysh PN. "Clinical Implications of Birth Trauma to the Brainstem and Upper Cervical Spine in Newborn Infants." *Proceedings from International Chiropractors Association Scientific Research Symposium*, Tampa, Fla., 1990.

7. Kent C, Gentempo P. "Sudden Infant Death Syndrome and Chiropractic." *ICA International Review of Chiropractic* 1992; Nov/Dec: 41–42.

8. Hospers LA, et al. Atlanto-Occipital Hypermobility in Sudden Infant Death Syndrome. *Today's Chiropractic* Jan/Feb, 1990 19(1); 36–40.

9. Towbin A. "Sudden Infant Death (cot death) Related to Spinal Injury." *Lancet* 1967;2:940.

10. Towbin A. "Latent spinal cord and brain stem injury in newborn infants." *Develop Med Child Neurol* 1969;11:54.

11. Sachis PN, et al. "The Vagus Nerve and Sudden Infant Death Syndrome: a morphometric study." *J Pediatrics* 1981; 98(2): 278.

12. Blakeslee S. "Crib death: Suspicion turns to the brain." *The New York Times.* Feb 14, 1989.

13. Flesia JM. "The vertebral subluxation complex part III-pathogenesis." *ICA International Review of Chiropractic* Nov/Dec 1992; 45–47.

14. Bonci A, Wynne C. "The Interface Between Sudden Infant Death Syndrome and Chiropractic." *Journal of Chiropractic Research* 1989; 5(3): 78.

15. Stiga J. "Sudden Infant Death Syndrome." *American Chiropractor* October 1983; 28.

16. Banks B, Beck R, Columbus M, et al. "Sudden Infant Death Syndrome: a literature review with chiropractic implications." *J Manip Physiol Ther* 1987; 10(5): 246.

17. Finnigan J. "Life Beyond Headaches." *Finnigan Clinic* 1307 Violet S.E., Olympia, WA 98503, 1999.

18. Schechtman VL, Lee MY, Wilson AJ, Harper RM. "Dynamics of respiratory patterning in normal infants and infants who subsequently died of the sudden infant death syndrome." *Pediatr Res* 1996 Oct;40(4):571–7.

19. Schechtman VL, Lee MY, Wilson AJ, Harper RM. Dynamics of respiratory patterning in normal infants and infants who subsequently died of the sudden infant death syndrome." *Pediatr Res* 1992 Jun;31(6): 606–12.

20. Schechtman VL, Harper RM, Kluge KA, Wilson AJ, Hoffman HJ, Southall DP. "Cardiac and respiratory patterns in normal infants and victims of the sudden infant death syndrome." *Sleep* 1988 Oct;11(5):413–24.

21. Wilson AJ, Southall DP. "Correlations between cardiorespiratory measures in normal infants and victims of sudden infant death syndrome." *Sleep* 1990 Aug;13(4):304–17.

22. Schechtman VL, Harper RM, Kluge KA, Wilson AJ, Hoffman HJ, Southall DP. "Heart rate variation in normal infants and victims of the sudden infant death syndrome." *Early Hum Dev* 1989 Jun;19(3):167–81. Harper RM, Leake B, Hodgman JE,

23. Hoppenbrouwers T. "Developmental patterns of heart rate and heart rate variability during sleep and waking in normal infants and infants at risk for the sudden infant death syndrome." *Sleep* 1982;5(1):28–38.

24. Haddad GG, Walsh EM, Leistner HL, Grodin WK, Mellins RB. "Abnormal maturation of sleep states in infants with aborted sudden infant death syndrome." *Pediatr Res* 1981 Jul;15(7):1055–7.

25. Harper RM, Leake B, Hoffman H, Walter DO, Hoppenbrouwers T, Hodgman J, Sterman MB. "Periodicity of sleep states is altered in infants at risk for the sudden infant death syndrome." *Science* 1981 Aug 28;213(4511):1030–2.

26. Challamel MJ, Revol M, Leszczynski MC, Debilly G. "12-hour pattern of the waking state in the normal infant and in the infant who has survived the 'syndrome of sudden infant death.'" *Rev Electroencephalogr Neurophysiol Clin* 1981 Sep;11(1):28–36.

27. Harper RM, Frostig Z, Taube D, Hoppenbrouwers T, Hodgman JE. "Development of sleep-waking temporal sequencing in infants at risk for the Sudden Infant Death Syndrome." *Exp Neurol* 1983 Mar;79(3):821–9.

28. Coons S, Guilleminault C. "Motility and arousal in near miss sudden infant death syndrome." *J Pediatr* 1985 Nov;107(5):728–32.

29. Harper RM, Leake B, Hoppenbrouwers T, Sterman MB, McGinty DJ, Hodgman J. "Polygraphic studies of normal infants and infants at risk for the sudden infant death syndrome: heart rate and variability as a function of state." *Pediatr Res* 1978 Jul;12(7):778–85.

30. Kluge KA, Harper RM, Schechtman VL, Wilson AJ, Hoffman HJ, Southall DP. "Spectral analysis assessment of respiratory sinus arrhythmia in normal infants and infants who subsequently died of sudden infant death syndrome." *Pediatr Res* 1988 Dec;24(6):677–82.

31. Navelet Y, Payan C, Guilhaume A, Benoit O. "Nocturnal sleep organization in infants "at risk" for sudden infant death syndrome." *Pediatr Res* 1984 Jul;18(7):654–7.

32. Schechtman VL, Raetz SL, Harper RK, Garfinkel A, Wilson AJ, Southall DP, Harper RM. "Dynamic analysis of cardiac R-R intervals in normal infants and in infants who subsequently succumbed to the sudden infant death syndrome." *Pediatr Res* 1992 Jun;31(6):606–12.

33. Cornwell AC, Feigenbaum P, Kim A. "SIDS, abnormal nighttime REM sleep and CNS immaturity." *Neuropediatrics* 1998 Apr;29(2):72–9.

34. Schechtman VL, Harper RM. "The maturation of correlations between cardiac and respiratory measures across sleep states in normal infants." *Sleep* 1992 Feb;15(1):41–7.

35. Gould JB, Lee AF, Morelock S. "The relationship between sleep and sudden infant death." *Ann N Y Acad Sci* 1988;533:62–77.

36. Peirano P, Lacombe J, Flores R, Singh BB, Guidasci S, Monod N. "Transcutaneous

oxygen tension and apnea during sleep stages in normal infants and infants at risk for sudden infant death syndrome." *Rev Electroencephalogr Neurophysiol Clin* 1986 Dec;16(4):395–402.

37. Kahn A, Groswasser J, Rebuffat E, Sottiaux M, Blum D, Foerster M, Franco P, Bochner A, Alexander M, Bachy A, et al. "Sleep and cardiorespiratory characteristics of infant victims of sudden death: a prospective case-control study." *Sleep* 1992 Aug;15(4):287–92.

38. Cornwell AC, Laxminarayan S. "A sleep disturbance in high risk for SIDS infants." *J Sleep Res* 1993 Jun;2(2):110–114.

39. Palmer BJ. "Chiropractic Clinical Controlled Research." *WB Conkey Company*, Hamond, Indiana, 1951.

40. Leach, R. "Theories of Subluxation Pathophysiology. In The chiropractic theories—a synopsis of scientific research." *Baltimore:Williams and Wilkins* 1986.

41. Homewood A. "Neurodynamics of The Vertebral Subluxation." *Canadian Memorial Chiropractic College*, Toronto; 1963.

42. Korr,I. Sustained Sympathicotonia. In: Korr, I. ed. "The Neurobiological mechanisms in manipulative therapy." *New York: Plenum Press* 1978:229–68.

43. Grostic JD. "Dentate Ligament–Cord Distortion Hypothesis." *Chiro Research Journal* 1988; 1(1): 47–55.

44. Stephenson, R. "Chiropractic Textbook." *Privately published by R. Stephenson, Davenport, 1927.*

45. Spencer J. "The neuropathophysiological relationship between asymmetrical spinal proprioception and postural muscle asynergism." *13th Biomechanical Conference on the Spine.* Palmer College of Chiropractic-West, Sunnyvale, CA 1982.

46. Crowe HS, Kleinman T. "Upper Cervical Influence on the Reticular System." *The Upper Cervical Monograph* 1991 5(1): 12–14.

47. Sweat R, Sievert T. "Chiropractic and The Vertebral Arteries Part One of Two." *Today's Chiropractic*, Sept/Oct, 1984 45–48.

48. Sweat R, Sievert T. "Chiropractic and The Vertebral Arteries Part Two of Two." *Today's Chiropractic*, Nov/Dec, 1984 23–24.

49. Abbot K: "Foramen magnum and high cervical cord lesions simulating degenerative disease of the nervous system." *Ohio State Medical Journal* 1950; 46:645–647.

50. Emery J: "Kinking of the medulla in children with acute oedema and hydrocephalus and its relationship to the dentate ligament." *Journal of Neurol Neurosurg Psychitat* 1967; 30:267–268.

51. Walker DW. "Hypoxic inhibition of breathing and motor activity in the foetus and newborn." *Clin Exp Pharmacol Physiol* 1995 Aug;22(8): 533–6.

52. Gutmann G. "Blocked Atlantal Nerve Syndrome in Infants and Small Children." Originally published in *Manuelle Medizine*, Springer-Verlag, 1987. English translation published in *International Review of Chiropractic* July/Aug 1990 37–43.

53. Smith L. "The Children's Doctor." *MPI's Dynamic Chiropractic*, Oct 25,1991; 31.

54. Bonci A, Wynne C. "The Interface Between Sudden Infant Death Syndrome and Chiropractic." *Journal of Chiropractic Research* 1989;5(3):78.

55. Willinger M, James LS, Catz C. "Defining the Sudden Infant Death Syndrome (SIDS): Deliberations of an expert panel convened by the National Institute of Child Health and Human Development." *Pediatr Pathol* 1991; 11: 677–84.

56. Bergman A, Beckwith J, Ray C, et al. "Sudden Infant Death Syndrome." *Proceedings of the Second International Conference on the Causes of Sudden Death in infants.* Seattle: University of Washington Press, 1970: 14–22.

57. Guyton AC. Textbook of Medical Physiology. *Saunders Company.* Philadelphia, PA, 1986, p 204.

58. Towbin A. "Central nervous system damage in the human fetus and newborn infant. Mechanical and hypoxic injury incurred in the fetal-neonatal period." *Am O Dis Child* 119:529, 1970.

59. Lucena J., Cruz-Sanchez FF. "The Interest of the Neurological Tissue Preservation for the Investigation of Sudden Infant Death Syndrome." *Journal of Neural Transmission Suppl.* 39:193–205, 1993.

60. Orlowski JP, Nodar RH, Lonsdale D. "Abnormal Brainstem Auditory Evoked Potentials in Infants with Threatened Sudden Infant Death Syndrome." *Clevland Clinic Quarterly* 46(3)77–81, Fall 1979.

61. Guilleminault C, Ariagno RL, Forno LS, Nagel L, Baldwin R, Owen M. "Obstructive Sleep Apnea and Near-Miss for SIDS: I. Report of an Infant with Sudden Death." *Pediatrics* 63(6):837–843, June 1979.

62. Lemmi H, Lonsdale D, Miranda F, Nealis J, Hughes JR, Nodar R. "The Interrelationship between Sudden Infant Death Syndrome and Sleep Apnea Syndrome." *Clinical Electroencephalography* 12(1):15–20, 1981.

63. Summers CG, Parker JC, Jr. "The Brain Stem in Sudden Infant Death Syndrome: A Postmortem Survey." *American Journal of Forensic Medicine and Pathology* 2(2):121–127, June 1981.

64. Schulte FJ, Albani M, Schnizer H, Bentele K. "Neuronal Control of Neonatal Respiration–Sleep Apnea and the Sudden Infant Death Syndrome." *Neuropediatrics* 13:3–14, 1982.

65. Atkinson JB, Evans OB, Ellison RS, Netsky MG. "Ischemia of the Brain Stem as a Cause of Sudden Infant Death Syndrome." *Archives of Pathology and Laboratory Medicine* 108(4):341–342, April 1984.

66. Kinney HC, Burger PC, Harrel FE, Jr., Hudson RP. "Reactive Gliosis in the Medulla Oblongata of Victims of the Sudden Infant Death Syndrome." *Pediatrics* 72(2):181–187. 1983.

67. Baba N, Quattrochi JJ, Reiner CB, Adrion W, McBride PT, Yates AJ. "Possible Role of the Brain Stem in Sudden Infant Death Syndrome." *Journal of the American Medical Association* 249 (20):2789–2791, May 27, 1983.

68. Naeye RL. "Brain-Stem and Adrenal Abnormalities in the Sudden Infant Death Syndrome." *American Journal of Clinical Pathology* 66(3):526–530, Sept. 1976.

69. Orlowski JP, Lonsdale D, Nodar RH, Williams GW. "Brainstem Dysfunction in the Infant Apnea Syndrome." *Clinical Electroencephalography* 13(4):226–232, Oct. 1982.

70. Pettigrew AG, Rahilly PM. "Brainstem Auditory Evoked Responses in Infants at Risk of Sudden Infant Death." *Early Human Development* 11(2):99–111, July 1985.

71. Quattrochi JJ, McBride PT, Yates AJ. "Brainstem Immaturity in Sudden Infant Death Syndrome: A Quantitative Rapid Golgi Study of Dendritic Spines in 95 Infants." *Brain Research* 325(1-2):39–48, Jan. 28, 1985.

72. Pauli RM et al. "Apnea and Sudden Unexpected Death in Infants with Achondroplasia." *Journal of Pediatrics* 104(3):342–348, Mar. 1984.

73. Takashima S, Armstrong D, Becker L, Bryan C. "Cerebral Hypoperfusion in the

Sudden Infant Death Syndrome?" Brainstem Gliosis and Vasculature. *Annals of Neurology* 4(3):257–262, Sept. 1978.

74. Bland JD, Emery JL. "Unexpected Death of Children with Achondroplasia after the Perinatal Period." *Developmental Medicine and Child Neurology* 24(4):489–492, Aug. 1982.

75. Nodar RH, Lonsdale D, Orlowski JP. "Abnormal Brain Stem Potentials in Infants with Threatened Sudden Infant Death Syndrome." *Otolaryngology and Head and Neck Surgery* 88 (5): 819–821, Sept/Oct. 1980.

76. Harrison H. Jr. "Infant Apnea Syndromes: Part II." *Alaska Medicine* 27(3):64–66, July–Sept. 1985.

77. Kinney H, Filiano JJ. "Brainstem Research in Sudden Infant Death Syndrome." *Pediatrician* 15(4):240–250, Sept. 1988.

78. Gottlieb, MS. "Neglected Spinal Cord, Brain Stem and Musculoskeletal Injuries Stemming From Birth Trauma." *J Manipulative Physiol Ther* Oct 1993;16(8): 537–543.

79. Korbkin R, Guilleminault C. "Neurologic Abnormalities in Near Miss for Sudden Infant Death Syndrome Infants." *Pediatrics* 64(3):369–374, Sept. 1979.

80. Ackland GL, Noble R, Hanson MA. "Red Nucleus Inhibits Breathing during Hypoxia in Neonates." *Respir Physiol* 1997 Nov;110(2–3):251–60.

81. Filiano JJ, Kinney HC. "Arcuate Nucleus Hypoplasia in the Sudden Infant Death Syndrome." *J Neuropathol Exp Neurol* 1992;51:394–403.

82. Speransky AD. "A Basis for the Theory of Medicine." *New York: International Publishers*, 1935.

83. Brown S. "Neurological Sequelae of Mechanoreceptor Deafferentation or Subluxation Complex." *Atlas Orthogonal Advanced Seminar*, Oct 1993.

84. Carpenter M. "Core Text of Neuroanatomy Third Edition." *Williams and Willkins Baltimore*, MA 1985

85. White and Panjabi. "Clinical Biomechanics of the Spine." Philadelphia. *Lippincott*, 1978, page 66.

86. Sweat RW. Atlas Orthogonal Procedures Advanced Seminar, Granby, Quebec Sept, 1999.

87. Seletz E. "Whiplash Injuries; Neurophysiological basis for pain and methods used for rehabilitation." *JAMA* 1958 Nov; 168 (13): 1750–5.

88. Pamphlett R, Raisanen J, Kum-Jew S. "Vertebral artery compression resulting from head movement: a possible cause of the sudden infant death syndrome." *Pediatrics* 1999 Feb; 103(2): 460–8.

89. Pamphlett R, Murray N: "Vulnerability of the infant brain stem to ischemia: a possible cause of sudden infant death syndrome." *J Child Neurol* 1996 May; 11(3): 181–4.

90. Saternus KS, Adam G. "Sudden infant death. Postmortem flow measurements in the large vessels of the neck for the demonstration of posture-dependent cerebral hypoxemia." *Dtsch Med Wochenschr* 1985 Feb 22; 110(8): 297–303.

91. Li YK, Zhang YK, Lu CM, Zhong SZ. "Changes and implications of blood flow velocity of the vertebral artery during rotation and extension of the head." *J Manipulative Physiol Ther* Feb1999; 22(2):91–5.

92. Jargiello T, Pietura R, Rakowski P, Szczerbo-Trojanowska M, Szajner M, Janczarek M Power. "Doppler imaging in the evaluation of extracranial vertebral artery compression

in patients with vertebrobasilar insufficiency." *Eur J Ultrasound* 1998 Dec;8(3): 149–56.

93. Johnson CP, How T, Scraggs M, West CR, Burns J. "A biomechanical study of the human vertebral artery with implications for fatal arterial injury." *Forensic Sci Int* 2000 Apr 10;109(3):169–182.

94. Deeg KH, Alderath W, Bettendorf U. "Basilar artery insufficiency—a possible cause of sudden infant death? Results of a Doppler ultrasound study of 39 children with apparent life-threatening events." *Ultraschall Med* 1998 Dec;19(6):250–8.

CHAPTER FIVE

1. Schechtman VL, Lee MY, Wilson AJ, Harper RM. "Dynamics of respiratory patterning in normal infants and infants who subsequently died of the sudden infant death syndrome." *Pediatr Res* 1996 Oct; 40(4):571–7.

2. Sweat RW. Atlas Orthogonal Placement, Basic III (Leg Check and Table Placement), 1981, Atlanta, GA.

3. Sweat RW. Atlas Orthogonal Chiropractic, Basic I (X-Ray Placement), 1981, Atlanta, GA.

4. Sweat RW. Atlas Orthogonal Chiropractic, Basic II (X-Ray Analysis, 1981, Atlanta, GA.

5. Sweat RW. Atlas Orthogonal Chiropractic, Basic IV (Instrument Adjusting), 1981, Atlanta, GA.

CHAPTER SIX

1. The SIDS Alliance. "Differentiating Between Sudden Infant Death Syndrome, Shaken Baby Syndrome, and Accidental Infant Deaths Associated With Bedsharing." Media Advisory, November 29, 1999.

2. Neel SS. "Whiplash – Atlanto-Axial Trauma." *MPI'S Dynamic Chiropractic*, October 15, 1989; 34.

3. Klougart N, Nilsson N, Jacobsen J. "Infantile Colic Treated by Chiropractors: A Prospective Study of 316 Cases." *J Manipulative Physiol Ther* 1989; 12(4): 281–8.

4. Pluhar GR, Schobert PD. "Vertebral Subluxation and Colic: A Case Study." *J Chiro Research and Clin Invest* 1991; 7(3):75–6.

5. Nilson N. "Infant Colic and Chiropractic." *Eur J Chiropractic* 1985; 33(4): 264–265.

6. Wiberg JMM, Nordsteen J, Nilsson N. "The Short-Term Effect of Spinal Manipulation in the Treatment of Infantile Colic: A Randomized Controlled Clinical Trial with a Blinded Observer." *J Manipulative Physiol Ther* 1999;22:517–22.

CHAPTER SEVEN

1. Mantero E, Crispini L. "Static Alterations of the Pelvic, Sacral, Lumbar Area due to Pregnancy, Chiropractic Treatment." World Chiropractic Conference 1982, Venice, Italy 59–68.

2. Fallon J. "Chiropractic and Pregnancy – A Partnership for the Future." *Int Rev Chiro.* 1990 Nov/Dec. 39–42.

3. Larsen JS, Pedersen OD, Ipsen L. "Induction of labor when a large fetus is suspected." *Ugeskr Laeger* 1991 Jan 14;153(3):181–3.

4. Butler J, Abrams B, Parker J, Roberts JM, Laros RK Jr. "Supportive nurse-midwife care is associated with a reduced incidence of cesarean section." *Am J Obstet Gynecol* 1993 May;168(5):1407–13.

5. Dierker LJ Jr, Rosen MG, Thompson K, Debanne S, Linn P. "The midforceps: maternal and neonatal outcomes." *Am J Obstet Gynecol* 1985 May 15;152(2):176–83.

6. Lieberman E, Lang JM, Frigoletto F Jr, Richardson DK, Ringer SA, Cohen A. "Epidural analgesia, intrapartum fever, and neonatal sepsis evaluation." *Pediatrics* 1997 Mar;99(3):415–9.

7. Lieberman E, Lang J, Richardson DK, Frigoletto FD, Heffner LJ, Cohen A. "Intrapartum maternal fever and neonatal outcome." *Pediatrics* 2000 Jan;105(1 Pt 1):8–13.

8. Lieberman E, Cohen A, Lang J, Frigoletto F, Goetzl L. "Maternal intrapartum temperature elevation as a risk factor for cesarean delivery and assisted vaginal delivery." *Am J Public Health* 1999 Apr;89(4):506–10.

9. Lieberman E, Lang JM, Cohen A, D'Agostino R Jr, Datta S, Frigoletto FD Jr. "Association of epidural analgesia with cesarean delivery in nulliparas." *Obstet Gynecol* 1996 Dec;88(6):993–1000.

10. Lieberman E. "No free lunch on labor day. The risks and benefits of epidural analgesia during labor." *J Nurse Midwifery* 1999 Jul–Aug;44(4):394–8.

11. The Bradley Method, Student Workbook, The American Academy of Husband-Coached Childbirth, Sherman Oaks, CA 1989.

CHAPTER EIGHT

1. Mortenson D. "Sudden Infant Death Syndrome." *Vector* Spring 2000; 2(5): 11.